NEONATAL ORTHOPAEDICS

NEONATAL ORTHOPAEDICS

Second Edition

N De Mazumder MBBS MS

Ex-Professor and Head
Department of Orthopaedics
Ramakrishna Mission Seva Pratishthan
Vivekananda Institute of Medical Sciences
Kolkata, West Bengal, India

Visiting Surgeon
Department of Orthopaedics
Chittaranjan Sishu Sadan
Kolkata, West Bengal, India

Ex-President
West Bengal Orthopaedic Association
(A Chapter of Indian Orthopaedic Association)
Kolkata, West Bengal, India

Consultant Orthopaedic Surgeon
Park Children's Centre
Kolkata, West Bengal, India

Foreword
AK Das

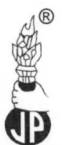

JAYPEE BROTHERS MEDICAL PUBLISHERS (P) LTD.

New Delhi • London • Philadelphia • Panama

Jaypee Brothers Medical Publishers (P) Ltd.

Headquarters
Jaypee Brothers Medical Publishers (P) Ltd.
4838/24, Ansari Road, Daryaganj
New Delhi 110 002, India
Phone: +91-11-43574357
Fax: +91-11-43574314
Email: jaypee@jaypeebrothers.com

Overseas Offices

J.P. Medical Ltd.
83, Victoria Street, London
SW1H 0HW (UK)
Phone: +44-2031708910
Fax: +02-03-0086180
Email: info@jpmedpub.com

Jaypee-Highlights Medical Publishers Inc.
City of Knowledge, Bld. 237, Clayton
Panama City, Panama
Phone: +507-301-0496
Fax: +507-301-0499
Email: cservice@jphmedical.com

Jaypee Brothers Medical Publishers Ltd.
The Bourse
111, South Independence Mall East
Suite 835, Philadelphia, PA 19106, USA
Phone: +267-519-9789
Email: joe.rusko@jaypeebrothers.com

Jaypee Brothers Medical Publishers (P) Ltd.
17/1-B, Babar Road, Block-B, Shaymali
Mohammadpur, Dhaka-1207
Bangladesh
Mobile: +08801912003485
Email: jaypeedhaka@gmail.com

Jaypee Brothers Medical Publishers (P) Ltd.
Shorakhute, Kathmandu
Nepal
Phone: +00977-9841528578
Email: jaypee.nepal@gmail.com

Website: www.jaypeebrothers.com
Website: www.jaypeedigital.com

© 2013, Jaypee Brothers Medical Publishers

All rights reserved. No part of this book may be reproduced in any form or by any means without the prior permission of the publisher.

Inquiries for bulk sales may be solicited at: jaypee@jaypeebrothers.com

This book has been published in good faith that the contents provided by the author contained herein are original, and is intended for educational purposes only. While every effort is made to ensure accuracy of information, the publisher and the author specifically disclaim any damage, liability, or loss incurred, directly or indirectly, from the use or application of any of the contents of this work. If not specifically stated, all figures and tables are courtesy of the author. Where appropriate, the readers should consult with a specialist or contact the manufacturer of the drug or device.

Neonatal Orthopaedics

First Edition: 2003
Second Edition: **2013**

ISBN 978-93-5090-372-8

Printed at Rajkamal Electric Press, Plot No. 2, Phase-IV, Kundli, Haryana.

Foreword

There has been a phenomenal breakthrough in the diagnosis and management of orthopaedic maladies in the last 50 years. This is partly because of introduction of newer alloys and different plastics in the construction of implants and orthosis, production of newer antibiotics, better understanding of biomechanics of bones and joints in the health and disease, and introduction of more efficient imaging techniques. Newer technology has advanced our horizon of knowledge, particularly, the advancement of information technology. Better methods of management of trauma with image intensifiers and better implants for fracture fixation, availability of various joint implants, advances in management of spinal injuries and deformities have vastly increased our capability to treat complicated abnormalities with much better functional results. Arthoscopic techniques have vastly improved the diagnosis of joint injuries and diseases with a minimum damage to joint structures and much early restoration of normal function.

As a result of these advances, it has become increasingly difficult for any individual surgeon to become expert in all the different techniques of surgery. Consequently, a number of subspecialties have emerged, e.g. Joint Replacement Surgery, Spinal Surgery, Arthroscopic Surgery, Paediatric Orthopaedics, Trauma Surgery and so on.

One of the subspecialties, which is getting popular, is paediatric orthopaedics. This deals with the diagnosis and management of diseases and injuries of bones, joints, muscles and nerves in children whose disease manifestations and management are quite different from adults. Neonatal orthopaedics is an offshoot of this specialty, which deals with the orthopaedic problems in neonates. Congenital deformities and abnormalities of muscles, bones and joints need to be diagnosed immediately or soon after birth in order to start treatment as early as possible. These need special awareness and expertise. Infections of bones and joints in the neonates pose special problems in diagnosis and management. Early effective treatment restores a normal anatomy and functions. Immediate correction of congenital deformities gives better correction before the structures get more rigid. This is comparatively a newer branch of orthopaedics, which is drawing the attention of some paediatric orthopaedicians. In our country, though paediatric orthopaedics is an established specialty, not many surgeons are yet interested to devote their attention to neonatal orthopaedic problems.

It is very encouraging that an experienced orthopaedic surgeon like Dr N De Mazumder has become interested in this new subspecialty and has written a book on this subject highlighting the special problems in orthopaedic affections in neonates. He had been the Professor and Head of orthopaedic service of a large hospital, such as Ramakrishna Mission Seva Pratishthan, Vivekananda Institute of Medical Sciences, Kolkata, West Bengal, India, which has also a large Obstetric Department. Consequently, he had the opportunity to study neonates also. He has written very lucidly with excellent diagrams covering the different aspects of this new specialty. I am sure that the book will be of great interest to orthopaedic surgeons, paediatric orthopaedic specialists as well as paediatricians.

AK Das
Ex-Professor
Department of Orthopaedics
Nil Ratan Sircar Medical College and Hospital
Kolkata, West Bengal, India

Ex-Emeritus Professor
BC Roy Polio Clinic and Hospital for Crippled Children
Kolkata, West Bengal, India

Ex-President
West Bengal Orthopaedic Association
(A Chapter of Indian Orthopaedic Association)
Kolkata, West Bengal, India

Preface to the Second Edition

Nine years from now, this book *Neonatal Orthopaedics* was published as a venture to bring in a new subject with descriptions of orthopaedic conditions in the neonatal period. Presently, the revised edition is being published. The first edition of this book published by M/s Jaypee Brothers Medical Publishers (P) Ltd., New Delhi, India, has been reviewed by Indian Journal of Orthopaedics in the April 2003 issue of the journal; a few lines are being coined here from Dr Ashok Kumar's review. This book is timely and has fulfilled a need of having a single source of information on neonatal orthopaedic problems and will serve as an important reference for the practicing orthopaedicians as well as the paediatricians. There is a wealth of information contained in this book. Overall, this book makes an interesting reading and will be a valuable addition to any medical library and is strongly recommended for postgraduate students, orthopaedicians, neonatologists and paediatricians.

The research, in the field of neonatal orthopaedics, has yet to get a momentum as many of the neonatal orthopaedic conditions have not been explored even today. Newer antenatal and natal diagnostic facilities are evolving with time. An effort is made to describe the diagnostic points to achieve a neonatal diagnosis. As written in the preface of the first edition, the details of surgical technique of the operations necessary for the correction of the neonatal deformities were avoided as the operations described were mostly undertaken long after the neonatal period.

All the 45 chapters with addition of keywords with each chapter, have been reviewed thoroughly with some illustrations added to bring out an effect of clarity of the conditions described. I am indebted to Professor Niloy Kanti Das for providing me with some clinical photographs. As this book has fulfilled to some extent, the need of postgraduate students, I have purposely kept it in an abridged form without much elaboration. The book *Essentials of Paediatric Orthopaedics* edited by me and published by M/s Jaypee Brothers Medical Publishers in 2007 has covered the paediatric orthopaedic conditions in a greater detail with an eye to present the readers, a comprehensive discussion on the subject. In the two books *Neonatal Orthopaedics* and *Essentials of Paediatric Orthopaedics*, I have tried to bring in the management of paediatric orthopaedic disorders from their onset in utero to the fully grown condition. My sincere thanks go to the M/s Jaypee Brothers Medical Publishers (P) Ltd., New Delhi, India.

N De Mazumder

Preface to the First Edition

The orthopaedic problems of the infants in their early days fascinate me for a long time. An involvement in orthopaedic practice, especially in paediatric orthopaedics, for more than three decades has led me to think about an early diagnosis of the orthopaedic conditions in the neonatal period, i.e. within 4 weeks of birth; which gives the opportunity for proper management of the condition and a better prognosis. The paediatric involvement stimulated me to study the orthopaedic conditions in the neonatal period in a greater detail.

Deviation from the normal growth of a baby in the mother's womb is considered as a defect or a disease. As the subject embryology deals with the anatomical study of the growth of the fetus, it needs proper study for an effective care of the newborn. Mention of embryology and growth of the fetal limbs is found in the *Charaka Samhita*—the famous ancient treatise in the Ayurveda. The care of the newborn is a well-known practice from the ancient times and has been outlined by Soranus (98-138 AD) of Ephesus. Weakness at birth was attributed to prematurity or an inheritance from infirm parents. A fetus, comfortable in the warm ambience of the mother's womb needs proper neonatal care of maintenance of body temperature and nutrition for the growth of the baby. The high rate of infant mortality in yesteryears was because of improper infant care after birth and from prematurity with its inevitability of suffering of the baby from a serious illness. The decline in the rate of infant mortality is an outcome of fervid elaboration of the subject neonatal medicine with an improvement in the care of the prematures and also of a normal baby.

The book deals with the orthopaedic conditions in the neonatal period. An effort is made to describe the diagnostic points to achieve a neonatal diagnosis. Many of the congenital orthopaedic conditions need their management to be started in the neonatal period to achieve better results. The misconception of starting the treatment of many congenital conditions after two or three years of age, when the limbs of the baby grow bigger, prevails today. It will not be an overstatement if I say, proper management of orthopaedic conditions in the neonatal period prevents secondary changes in the bones of the deformed parts. The management becomes easier with the use of splint or brace after birth, which is recommended in the book. The details of surgical technique of the operations necessary for the correction of the neonatal deformities are purposely avoided in this monograph, as they are mostly undertaken long after the neonatal period.

The book, with a new approach without much elaboration, may arouse interest of the general orthopaedic surgeons who treat children, neonatologists, paediatricians and the paediatric orthopaedic surgeons. I have tried to cover as many neonatal orthopaedic conditions as possible. I would like to apologize to the readers for any inadvertent omission.

I am grateful to Mr Shambhu N Pal, Librarian and Head, Sudhira Memorial Library, Chittaranjan National Cancer Institute, Kolkata, West Bengal, India, for his meticulous care and help extended during preparation for publication of the book. To M/s Jaypee Brothers Medical Publishers (P) Ltd, New Delhi, India, my sincere thanks go for publishing the book and to Dr Prasanta Pujari, Mrs Gouri Sen and Mr Biswanath Mukherjee, for the photographs of the book, I owe my special thanks. My sincere thanks are due to the Secretary, the Dean, my colleagues in the Department of Orthopaedics, to name specially Dr Tapas Chakraborty and Dr Chandrachur Bhattacharya, the Department of Paediatrics, the Department of Genetics, the Department of Radiology and other participating departments of the Ramakrishna

Mission Seva Pratishthan, Vivekananda Institute of Medical Sciences, Kolkata, West Bengal, India, where I carried out major part of this work during my tenure of service of long 35 years.

I sincerely acknowledge the active participation and help of the sisters, splint-makers and other staff of the Department of Orthopaedics for the successful completion of the work.

I am indebted to Professor AK Das, the pioneer in paediatric orthopaedics in Eastern India, who took particular care to go through the manuscript and enriched me with a Foreword.

I gratefully acknowledge the help of Dr Niloy Kanti Das, Orthopaedic Surgeon, attached to the Institute of Child Health, Kolkata, West Bengal, India, by providing illustrations of some of his patients (Figs 6.3, 10.1, 10.2, 10.3, 19.2, 21.1 and 21.2).

My thanks and gratitude are due to the parents of my large number of patients, whose helpful participation was key to the successful completion of this work. The line drawings of the pictures in the book have been done by me and the cover design by my beloved daughter, Jayasmita. To my wife, Swapna and to my son-in-law, Sandipan, I owe my special thanks for their various help during the preparation of this book.

N De Mazumder

Contents

SECTION 1: GENERAL ASPECTS OF NEONATAL ORTHOPAEDICS

1. **Importance of Neonatal Orthopaedics as a Subject** — 1
   - *Perspectives in Neonatology* 1
   - *Care of the Newborn* 1
   - *Care and Feeding of Premature Infants* 2

2. **Anatomical and Physiological Consideration of a Neonate** — 5
   - *A Baby in the Mother's Womb* 5
   - *The Growth and Development of a Neonate* 6
   - *Physiological Functions of a Newborn Baby* 7

3. **Antenatal Diagnosis of Orthopaedic Conditions** — 9
   - *Detection of Musculoskeletal Abnormalities in the Neonatal Period* 9

4. **Importance of Genetics in Neonatal Orthopaedic Diseases** — 13
   - *Incidence of Genetic Disorders among Neonates* 13
   - *Abnormality of Genes Causing Genetic Disorders* 13
   - *Inherited Neonatal Orthopaedic Conditions* 14
   - *Cause of Genetic Disorders* 15

5. **Congenital Malformations** — 16
   - *Congenital Malformations* 16

6. **General Abnormalities of Skeletal Development, Evident at Birth** — 19
   - *Dwarfism Presenting at Birth* 19
   - *Signs of Dwarfism at Birth in Different Diseases* 19

7. **Disorders of Voluntary Muscles Presenting at Birth** — 33
   - *Congenital Muscular Dystrophy* 33
   - *Congenital Structural Myopathies* 34
   - *Myotonia Congenita (Thomsen Disease)* 34
   - *Congenital Myotonic Dystrophy* 35
   - *Infantile Spinal Muscular Atrophy* 35

8. **Can We Diagnose Cerebral Palsy in the Neonatal Period?** — 36
   - *Cerebral Palsy* 36

9. **Birth Injuries** — 38
   - *Head and Neck Injuries* 38
   - *Cephalhaematoma* 38

- Caput Succedaneum 39
- Intra-cranial Haemorrhage 39
- Birth Fractures 39
- Epiphyseal Separation 41
- Birth Injuries of the Brachial Plexus 41

10. **Congenital Developmental Anomalies of the Extremities in the Neonate** 44
    - Etiology 44
    - Classification of Limb Deficiencies 46
    - Congenital Constriction Band Syndrome (Streeter Syndrome) 47

11. **Neonatal Rickets** 49
    - Etiology 49
    - Clinical, Biochemical and Radiographic Features 49
    - Management 50

SECTION 2: LOWER LIMB ANOMALIES

12. **Bent Bones in a Neonate** 51
    - Congenital Kyphoscoliosis Tibia and Fibula 51

13. **Congenital Pseudoarthrosis of the Tibia and Fibula** 54
    - Congenital Pseudoarthrosis of Tibia 54
    - Congenital Pseudoarthrosis of Fibula 55

14. **Congenital Lower Limb Defects** 56
    - Congenital Defects of the Femur 56
    - Congenital Longitudinal Deficiency of the Tibia 57
    - Congenital Longitudinal Deficiency of the Fibula 59

15. **Proximal Femoral Focal Deficiency** 63
    - Classification 64
    - Management 64

16. **Congenital Coxa Vara** 66
    - Pathology 66
    - Clinical Findings 66
    - Radiographic Features 67
    - Diagnosis 68
    - Treatment 68

17. **Foetal Development and Natural History of Lower Limb Rotation** 71
    - Version 71

18. **Postural and Congenital Deformities of the Foot and Ankle** 73
    - Metatarsus Adductus Versus Congenital Metatarsus Varus 73
    - Congenital Talipes Calcaneovalgus 74

- Congenital Convex Pes Valgus at Birth 74
- Neonatal Deformities of the Toes 76

19. **Club Foot**   78
    - Club Foot 78

20. **Arthrogryposis Multiplex Congenita**   88
    - Arthrogryposis Multiplex Congenita 88
    - Other Forms of Arthrogryposis 93

21. **Congenital Subluxations and Dislocations Around the Knee**   96
    - Congenital Dislocation of the Patella 98

22. **Developmental Dysplasia of the Hip**   100
    - Developmental Dysplasia of the Hip 100

23. **Congenital Abduction Contracture of the Hip and Pelvic Obliquity**   111
    - Clinical and Radiological Features 111
    - Treatment 111
    - Prognosis 112

SECTION 3: VERTEBRAL ANOMALIES

24. **Vertebral Agenesis, Fusions and the Fusion Defects**   113
    - Development of Vertebral Bodies 113
    - Vertebral Agenesis 115

25. **Congenital Scoliosis**   117
    - Congenital Scoliosis 117

26. **Klippel-Feil Syndrome**   119
    - Etiology 119
    - Clinical Features 119
    - Treatment 119

27. **Congenital Muscular Torticollis**   121
    - Cause 121
    - Clinical Features 121
    - Treatment 122

SECTION 4: UPPER LIMB AND SHOULDER GIRDLE ANOMALIES

28. **Congenital High Scapula (Sprengel's Shoulder)**   123
    - Etiology 123
    - Clinical Features 123
    - Diagnosis 123

29. **Congenital Pseudoarthrosis of the Clavicle**   125
   - *Etiology 125*
   - *Clinical Findings 125*
   - *Diagnosis 125*

30. **Cleidocranial Dysostosis and Congenital Absence of the Pectoral Muscles**   127
   - *Cleidocranial Dysostosis 127*
   - *Congenital Absence of the Pectoral Muscles 128*

31. **Congenital Radioulnar Synostosis and Congenital Synostosis of the Elbow**   129
   - *Congenital Radioulnar Synostosis 129*
   - *Congenital Synostosis of the Elbow 130*

32. **Radial Club Hand and Congenital Longitudinal Deficiency of the Ulna**   131
   - *Radial Club Hand Deformity 131*
   - *Congenital Longitudinal Deficiency of the Ulna 134*

33. **Hand and Finger Affections, Present at Birth**   136
   - *Syndactyly 137*
   - *Polydactyly 137*
   - *Congenital Longitudinal Deficiency of the Thumb 138*
   - *Miscellaneous Finger Deformities 139*
   - *Congenital Clasped Thumb 139*
   - *Congenital Trigger Thumb 140*
   - *Hand-reduction Malformations 140*

SECTION 5: NEONATAL INFECTIONS

34. **Neonatal Osteomyelitis**   142
   - *Neonatal Osteomyelitis 142*

35. **Acute Psoas Abscess in a Newborn Infant**   148
   - *Acute Psoas Abscess 148*

SECTION 6: MISCELLANEOUS CONDITIONS

36. **Mucolipidoses**   150
   - *Gangliosidosis Type I 150*
   - *Mucolipidosis II (I-cell disease) 150*

37. **Neonatal Tetanus**   152
   - *Neonatal Tetanus 152*

38. **Syndromes with Skeletal Problems, Present at Birth**   153
   - *Down Syndrome 153*
   - *Marfan Syndrome 154*

- *Walker-Warburg Syndrome* 154
- *Meckel Syndrome* 154
- *Ellis-Van Creveld Syndrome* 155
- *Velo-cardio-facial Syndrome* 155
- *Smith-Lemli-Pitz Syndrome* 155
- *Widervanck or Cervico-oculo-acoustic Syndrome* 155
- *Oral-facial-digital Syndrome* 155
- *Goldenhar Syndrome* 155
- *Treacher Collins Syndrome (Mandibulo-facial Dysostosis)* 155
- *Möbius Syndrome* 156
- *Early Amnion Disruption Syndrome* 156
- *Scalp Defect—Ectrodactyly Syndrome or Adams-Oliver Syndrome* 156
- *Cornelia de Lange's or Brachmann de Lange Syndrome* 156
- *Thrombocytopenia-absent Radius Syndrome* 156
- *Asphyxiating Thoracic Dystrophy (Jeune Syndrome)* 156
- *Rubinstein-Taybi Syndrome* 156
- *Beckwith-Wiedemann Syndrome* 156

39. Neonatal Gangrene   158
- *Neonatal Gangrene* 158

40. Rheumatic Disorders Manifesting in the Neonatal Period   160
- *Systemic Lupus Erythematosus* 160

41. Neonatal Malignancy and Sacrococcygeal Teratoma   161
- *Neonatal Malignancy* 161
- *Sacrococcygeal Teratoma* 162

42. Conjoined (Siamese) Twins   163
- *Conjoined (Siamese) Twins* 163

43. Caffey's Disease   166
- *Caffey's Disease* 166

44. Syndromes having Craniosynostosis Presenting at Birth   168
- *Craniosynostosis* 168

45. Chondrodysplasia Punctata   170
- *Severe Rhizomelic Type* 170
- *Conradi-Hunermann Type* 170

Index   173

Section 1: General Aspect of Neonatal Orthopaedics

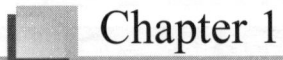

Chapter 1

Importance of Neonatal Orthopaedics as a Subject

> **Keywords:** Better care of neonates by neonatologists, special care and feeling of premature, necessity of an incubator are essential in neonatal management.

Since Alexander J Schaffer[1] coined the word "neonatology" about six decades ago, the subject neonatology, which deals with a baby's (neonate's) extrauterine progress for the first-four weeks after birth, has reached a fascinating height of development.

PERSPECTIVES IN NEONATOLOGY

The highly interesting subject of neonatal orthopaedics can be studied only when we discuss the development of neonatology.

High infant mortality rate, a perpetual problem of the yesteryears, continued in the late eighteenth century despite introduction of artificial feeding in the Paris Foundling Hospital. Care of the infants under a physician was not a practice even as late as the middle of the nineteenth century. Further more, home delivery system was the method widely practised in Europe because of non-establishment of lying-in hospitals. The high maternal mortality rate from puerperal fever was a stimulus for the improvement of hospital standard with a rise in the number of skilled obstetricians. With the increase in number of hospital deliveries in the newly established lying-in hospitals, the care of the neonates had fallen in the hands of the specialised physicians. Thus, the field of neonatology emerged at about 1950, when a number of paediatricians, better known as neonatologists got interested in the study of the infants within four weeks of life, not only to reduce the high rate of infant mortality, specially among the prematures, but also to know about the pathogenesis of the diseases from which the infants were suffering from the intrauterine life.

CARE OF THE NEWBORN

Salting and swaddling of the newborn infants had been practised until only a century ago since these were first advocated by Soranus[2] (AD 98-138) of Ephesus. The practice of testing the quality of breast milk is in vogue from his time. The old idea of keeping the baby free from crookedness or becoming a lame by swaddling was nullified by William Cadogan[3] (1711-97). The cause of weakness of nowborn babies was considered to be due to prematurity or from infirm parents. The standard birth-weight of a baby was not known till 1815 when based on recorded birth weights of 7077 newborn infants a report was published from the Maternite hospital in Paris.

CARE AND FEEDING OF PREMATURE INFANTS

The programme of improving the standard of infant care with an eye to achieve a decline in the infant mortality rate continued. France, the pioneer in this respect, specially in establishing modern, organized maternity and infant hygiene programme brought in improvement in child care for the premature babies. Budin,[4] the head of the Obstetric department at Charite and Maternite hospitals in Paris first felt the importance of three cardinal points of maintenance of infants' body temperature, proper feeding of the baby and the susceptibility of the premature of various diseases. Thus, the necessity of an incubator was first felt.

The famous story of Licetus Fortunio, who was born as a foetus of 5" length is known to many. He was brought to Jerome Bardi and other physicians of Rapalio by his father in living condition. His father used his medical knowledge and observations from nature and put the foetus in an oven where the heat was measured by a thermometer, and succeeded in rearing him and increased the growth of the baby.

This stimulated Johann Georg von Ruehl[5] to be instrumental in the manufacture of a double-walled metal incubator in 1835. These incubators were modified with time and the care of the infants improved. The mortality rate of the prematures fell significantly.

In 1893, Budin introduced special unit for the prematures. Julius H. Hess[6] (1876-1955) founded the first centre for the premature babies in USA at the Michael Ruse Hospital in Chicago utilizing this experience from his study in Germany and Austria.

Diagnosis of prematurity from birth weight was introduced by Alexandra Gueniot[7] in 1872. But after about eight decades in 1948 World Health Assembly adopted a birth weight of 2500 gm or less as an international definition of prematurity. A decade later, the concept of premature babies was changed to low birth weight babies by an expert committee of WHO.

The intrauterine growth of the baby with respect to gestation was standardised and published by Lubchenco et al[8] in 1963 and they had categorised AGA as the average size of the baby for the gestational age, SGA the small sized and LGA the large sized baby. Apgar score on the size of the newborn babies was introduced accordingly. Neonatal mortality depended much on the weight of the baby.

The importance of feeding the low birth weight infant gained importance, as a result. Various types of milk other than the breast milk were introduced at different times starting from butter milk, skimmed milk with added carbohydrate and albumin milk. JPC Griffith[9] in 1912 opined that the breast-fed babies have five times more chances of survival. Prior to this Abraham Jacob[10] in 1873 first proposed boiling of milk. On the contrary various authors showed that the infants had difficulty in digesting casein and/or fat.

The effort continued to improve the survival rate of the premature babies. While early infant feeding was advocated by some authors, other recommended late feeding. Because the infants cannot stand starvation they should be first fed at twelve hours from birth was opined by Hess. The other school of thought about delayed feeding as the swallowing process was imperfect in premature babies and hence the chance of aspiration pneumonia. The method of delayed feeding after about 36 to 48 hours was started in USA first and then in UK. The latter method was questioned by YIppo[11] of Finland in early twentieth Century. Various studies showed adverse reports with high incidence of infant mortality and development of disabilities among babies, specially spastic diplegia because of undernutrition. The effect was further grave because of lesser growth of many organs, increase of neurologic handicap and mental defects.

Small piece and Dabies[12] in 1964 reported that early milk feeding reduced hypoglycaemia, neonatal jaundice and hyponatraemia in premature infants. The method was well-established in 1970.

Importance of Neonatal Orthopaedics as a Subject

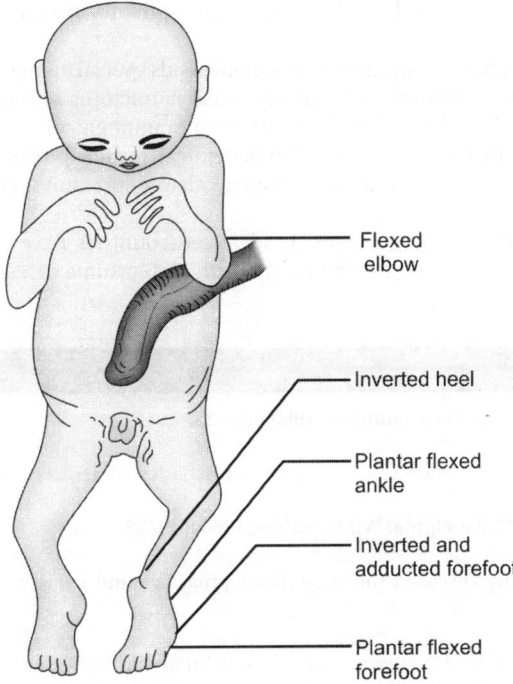

Fig. 1.1: Normal foetal posture at birth

Various methods of feeding was introduced from time to time as the premature baby suffered from suckling. So, gavage or dropper feeding was introduced. Feeding by indwelling nasogastric tube was first reported by Royce et al[13] in 1951. Total intravenous alimentation using peripheral veins began at around 1970.

The infant mortality rate though much abated was a problem to the neonatologists because of newer types of infections affecting the infants, specially the premature babies. Budin and his associates showed four different sources—the skin, the umbilicus, the gastrointestinal and the respiratory tracts, for carrying infection and introduced various methods for the cure in special units for the premature.

Even today in a well-equipped modern hospital significant number of foetuses may be infected in utero and a number of neonates can acquire an infection at birth or in the first month of life. Why the newborn babies kept in intensive care units are not immune from sepsis, meningitis is yet unknown. Only explanation towards the cause, is the changing pattern of bacterial infection. However, mortality rate from neonatal sepsis has fallen considerably with the introduction of ICU with an overall improvement or salvation of the premature babies.

With the emergence of neonatology as a super speciality of paediatric, the orthopaedic diseases, specific for the neonatal period have been stressed and got proper importance. The treatment of various neonatal diseases is difficult because of the small size of the baby and still smaller size of the anatomical structures within. Normal foetal posture at birth (Fig. 1.1) shows a flexed attitude, which is continued temporarily in the neonatal period. Effort for improvement in the management of neonatal diseases has been witnessed from the early part of this century with the introduction of drawing of blood by different methods like a modified suction device, intraperitoneal injections of saline and rarely of glucose solution for the treatment of persistent diarrhoea. The method of transfusion of blood through the umbilical vein helped in the subsequent method of exchange transfusion for haemorrhagic diseases of the newborn.

Intragastric oxygen therapy was introduced by YIppo as early as 1917 to combat respiratory distress of the premature babies.

Iatrogenic diseases in neonates, although not many in number two of them needs special mentioning. Due to sulfisoxazole prophylaxis in early fifties to prevent bacterial infections kernicterus developed. Similarly "Gray syndrome" emerged as a distressing ailment from over use of chloramphenicol.

Neonatologists are now well equipped with different types of biochemical testing procedures, amniocentesis, ultrasonography, foetal monitoring, continuous positive airway pressure (cPAP), mechanical ventilation and other methods.

Despite such improvement, even today 10% surviving infants in advanced countries have major handicap like cerebral palsy. So, the infant care should begin long before birth and in some cases even before conception.

REFERENCES

1. Schaffer AJ. Diseases of the newborn. Philadelphia: WB Saunders; 1960.pp.1-25.
2. Soranus: Ibid.
3. Cadogan W. An Eassy upon Nursing, J. Roberts, London, 1748, quoted by Schaffer AJ, Diseases of the Newborn. Philadelphia: WB Saunders; 1960.
4. Budin: Schaffer AJ. Diseases of the Newborn. Philadelphia: WB Saunders; 1960.pp.1-25.
5. Von Ruehl JG:Ibid.
6. Hess JH. Book on Premature and Congenitally Diseased Infants. Philadelphia: Lea and Febiger; 1922, quoted by Schaffer AJ, 1960.
7. Gueniot A. Ibid.
8. Lubchenco LO, Hansman G, Dressler M, Boyd E. Intrauterine growth as estimated from liveborn birth weight data at 24 to 42 weeks of gestation. Pediatrics 1963;32: 793-800.
9. Griffith JPC. The ability of mothers to nurse their children. J Am Med Assoc 1912;59:1874.
10. Jacobi A. Schaffer AJ: Diseases of the Newborn. Philadelphia: WB Saunders; 1960.pp.1-25.
11. Ylppo: Ibid.
12. Smallpiece and Dabies: Lancet 1964;2:1939.
13. Royce, et al. Pediatrics 1951;8:79.

Chapter 2

Anatomical and Physiological Consideration of a Neonate

Keywords: Embryonic development, growth and development of a neonate and its various body parts.

A BABY IN THE MOTHER'S WOMB

Starting from a fertilised ovum, the development of a baby in the mother's womb takes place in two phases. The first phase is the embryonic phase of about two months, when the fertilised ovum multiplies from a single cell into different tissues and structures. The rest of the seven odd months is the time for the foetus to grow and mature into a fully formed baby. By and large the embryonic development follows a time frame and the embryo takes a recognisable human form by the end of the second month. After a little more than nine months of the onset of development as a fertilised ovum, a baby is born in an immature form and takes many months for the hands and feet to achieve maturity for adopting adult functions. The hands become chief tactile organs after many months and till then the lips are used for feeling. The locomotor activity of the lower limbs begins when the child learns walking at about one year of age.

The single cell of fertilised ovum divides and forms a cluster of cells known as the morula. The central cells of this mass, devoid of nutrition from the surface, forms cystic space and thus transforming into a blastocyst. The implantation into the uterine mucosa takes place at this stage, about nine days from the date of fertilisation. The outer layer of this blastocyst forms the ultimate placenta and soon becomes a syncytium known as trophoblast. The other cells within the blastocyst congregate at a place to form an inner cell mass, which is surrounded by a large cystic cavity known as extra-embryonic coelom. Two other cavities known as amnion and yolk sac develop within this inner cell mass separated by a mass of cells forming an embryonic plate. The tissues and organs of the embryo will differentiate from this plate. There are three types of cells in this embryonic plate, the ectodermal cells on the amniotic aspect and the endodermal cells towards the yolk sac part with the primary mesodermal cells in between.

The nervous system of the body develops from the ectodermal tissues—a groove on it transforming into a tube by the union of its edges forming the neural tube. A row of cells develops from the ectoderm towards the endoderm form the notochord. The neural tube and the notochord have alongside them the mesoderm in three long strips. The mesoderm nearest to the midline or the paraxial mesoderm is segmented into mesodermal somites. The somite producing the sclerotome surrounds the neural tube and notochord producing future vertebrae and dura mater; and the other cells of somite placed laterally from the myotome or muscle plate, which are the precursor of the muscles of the body wall.

The intermediate strip of mesoderm is again segmented and forms the intermediate cell mass projecting ventrally between the outer two strips. From this develops the future uro-genital system. The outer strip of mesoderm is unsegmented and is known as the lateral plate. The ventrally placed yolk sac is ultimately enclosed by the lateral plate and its mesoderm is split into two layers, the inner lining covering the yolk sac—becomes the future gut and an outer layer. In between the layers is the coelomic cavity.

The limb buds grow from the lateral plate mesoderm. The muscles of the upper limb migrate for a considerable distance to gain attachment to the trunk. The innervation once developed for a muscle remains the same even after migration; the examples are latissimus dorsi and trapezius. The limbs are connected to the trunk by means of bones of the pectoral and pelvic girdles. The muscles of the limb buds although develop from unsegmented lateral plate mesoderm, the nerve supply to them is from well arranged limb plexuses from the spinal cord with a definite segmental pattern.

THE GROWTH AND DEVELOPMENT OF A NEONATE

This depends much on its perinatal anatomical positions and physiological functions. An important nondevelopment is the unmedullated character of the cerebrospinal tracts. The foetal circulation also differs from adult circulation as the blood is oxygenated in the placenta and not in the lungs. Blood goes from venous circulation to the left and right heart both and then into the arterial stream bypassing the liver and the lungs through three structures—the ductus venosus, the foramen ovale and the ductus arteriosus. Both the sides of the heart, the right and the left, pump blood equally to the tissues and the placenta. The ductus venosus, placed between the layers of lesser omentum in the inferior surface of the liver, carries placental oxygenated blood directly to the inferior vena cava bypassing the capillaries of the liver. After birth, the non-functioning ductus venosus becomes a fibrous cord and is known as ligamentum venosus. The foramen ovale circulates blood directly to left atrium from the right one and is closed after birth leaving a shallow depression, the fossa ovalis. The stream of venous blood in the right atrium brought through the superior vena cava rarely mixes with the stream of oxygenated blood brought by the inferior vena cava, crosses it and enters the pulmonary trunk via the right ventricle. The non-functioning lungs are short circuited by the passage of blood from the pulmonary trunk through the ductus arteriosus into the aorta. The deoxygenated blood is circulated from the aorta through the umbilical arteries into the placenta for oxygenation. After birth ductus arteriosus becomes cord like and is known as ligamentum arteriosum. The circulation through the lungs is then established.

The features of the newborn in general show a better developed cranium and upper limbs than the pelvis and lower limbs. There is almost a non-existent neck with the chin touching the chest and the shoulder. The vertical height of the face is smaller than the horizontal length due to non-eruption of teeth and non-development of maxillary sinuses. The cheeks thus become prominent. The hand does not have any tactile sensation but the grasping reflex is very strong. Most of the viscera remains in the abdomen because of lesser development of the pelvis.

Some of the special features of the newborn need mentioning, as these help in the diagnosis of many diseases.

The Skull

The cranium is disproportionately large in comparison to the face. Where the box of the skull ossifies in cartilage, the vault of the skull and the face ossify in membrane and at birth are ossified but mobile on each other. The frontal, parietal, occipital and squamous part of temporal bone are attached by fibrous tissue and not by sutures as in the adult. The anterior and posterior fontanelles produced at the lines of separation of the bones in the midline of the vault are of clinical significance in detecting hydration of an infant. The posterior fontanelle closes by one year of age and the anterior by the second year; but clinically the anterior one is usually not palpable after the age of one and a half years. The bones of the vault are compact at birth and do not contain cancellous element with redbone marrow as in the adults.

The Face

At birth, the facial bones like the mandible is developed in two halves, joined together by fibrous joint in the midline (which ossifies at one year of the age of the baby), with the shallow, ill developed maxillae having developing teeth and rudimentary paranasal sinuses within them. The angle of the mandible is obtuse with the coronoid process placed at a higher level than the condyle. The blunt-tipped tongue is relatively large and cannot be protruded. The Eustachian orifices are at the same level with the high arched hard palate.

The Neck

The neck of the newborn being short the position of its viscera is at a higher level with the epiglottis and larynx lying nearer the base of the tongue. The left brachiocephalic vein is above the level of sternal notch while crossing the trachea; the latter and the larynx are of small bore.

The Thorax

The rib cage shows horizontal position of the ribs causing a short neck and a higher level of the diaphragm; the abdominal volume is thereby increased giving room to many viscera including the pelvic ones. The thymus is very large, occupies the neck, the superior and part of the anterior mediastinum.

The Abdomen

The size and shape of the viscera in the newborn are different from those in the adults. The liver is quite big; the surface of the kidney is lobulated; the suprarenal glands are very big. The pelvis is small and the fundus of the urinary bladder lies above the level of the symphysis pubis.

The Upper Limb

The upper limbs are better developed than the lower ones in the newborn; the growth in length occurs more at the shoulder and wrist than at the elbow.

The Lower Limb

The flexed and externally rotated foetal position of the lower limb remains for six months or more after birth. The limb has its maximum growth at the knee than at the hip or ankle.

The Vertebral Column

The C-shaped vertebral column at birth gains its curvature with the adoption of posture; necessary for sitting and walking. The spinal canal extends upto L3 vertebra at birth.

PHYSIOLOGICAL FUNCTIONS OF A NEWBORN BABY

The changes from the intrauterine life are observed as the baby has to breathe on his or her own due to establishment of his/her own circulation, independent from mother. The baby has to maintain his/her own body temperature and renal function.

Non-shivering thermogenesis and use of 'brown fat' in the generation of chemical heat are two distinct methods adopted by the infants to keep themselves warm.

The newborn's kidney is medullary organ regarding its function of enzyme maturation. The renal vascular resistance, like pulmonary vascular resistance is higher in the newborn and gradually becomes less and less. The renal perfusion is initially low after birth with a specially low renal threshold for bicarbonate ions.

Dawes and strang[1] elucidated establishment of an effective neonatal circulation from foetal circulation with the reduction of pulmonary resistance as an accompaniment of onset of respiration.

Barclay, Franklin and Prichard at the Nuffield Institute, Oxford studied post-partum closure of the ductus venosus, the ductus arteriosus and the foramen ovale by cineradiography.

Apgar and James[2] at Columbia found excess organic acids in cord blood as an evidence of transient intrauterine asphyxia in some stressed babies.

Respiratory functions were studied by famous physiologists like Henderson, Krogh, Hasselbach, Haldam, Bohr and Barcroft. Electromagnetic flow meters were used by Nicholas Assali[3] an obstetrician from Los Angeles for direct measurement of uterine and placental blood flow as early as 1950.

Instrumentation for the measurement of foetal heart rate by polarographic measurement of amniotic fluid was introduced by Quilligan and Hon[4] at New Haven and by Caldegro Barela[5] in South America three decades ago.

REFERENCES

1. Dawes, Straz. Quoted from Smith CA: Physiology of the Newborn Infant, 3rd edn. Springfield IV. Charles C Thomas, 1959.
2. Apgar, James Ibid.
3. Assali N. Ibid.
4. Quilligan, Hon Ibid.
5. Barela C Ibid.

Chapter 3

Antenatal Diagnosis of Orthopaedic Conditions

Keywords: Diagnostic methods to detect foetal malformatiions—due to chromosomal or environmental defects—detection of neonatal musculoskeletal defects by history taking, Apgar score, clinical examination and anthropometric measurement.

A foetus grows within the mother's womb in a definite pattern. Any change in this pattern will lead to congenital malformation. The change may be due to a change in the uterine environment or due to chromosomal defect. The limbs start growing from the 5th to 6th week of intrauterine life. Changes which develop prior to this period is due to chromosomal abnormality. The changes which take place after that period are due to environmental defect.

Therefore, to diagnose any congenital malformation in the antenatal period needs a detail maternal history taking which includes age of the patient, intake of different medicines, presence of diabetes, suffering of the mother from any infection during pregnancy, any trauma during pregnancy, maternal or foetal problems, if any, in the previous pregnancy. The assessment of foetal growth is done as it happens in three phases—the first 12 weeks of organogenesis, the next phase from 13 to 28 weeks and the third phase from 28 weeks onward upto 40 weeks when the foetus grows upto its fullest development. Various congenital malformations occur due to intake of drugs life thalidomide, as it happened in UK and also from maternal suffering from diabetes or infections like measles. Any defect anticipated from history should be corroborated by foetal diagnostic tests like amniocentesis, ultrasonography and others.

The intake of different medicines which cause foetal malformation are aminopterin, thalidomide (not used now-a-days), trimethadione, paramethadione and antibiotics like chloramphenicol and tetracycline. The latter causes retarded skeletal growth, hypoplasia of enamel and pigmentation of teeth.

Various diagnostic methods used to detect intrauterine foetal orthopaedic conditions are:
i. Amniography—to diagnose meningomyelocele
ii. Ultrasonography in the third trimester to diagnose cranial malformations and gestational age
iii. Amniocentesis for cytogenetic studies on foetus
iv. Chorionic venous sampling to detect Down syndrome and the like, and rarely X-ray examination (not in the first-two trimester) to know about bone dysplasias, skeletal malformation and fractures.

DETECTION OF MUSCULOSKELETAL ABNORMALITIES IN THE NEONATAL PERIOD

When an orthopaedic surgeon is asked to examine a newborn baby to detect the presence of any orthopaedic problem, the methods he should follow are:
1. To obtain a thorough history, which encompasses
   i. Antenatal history

ii. Natal history
   iii. Neonatal history
   iv. Family
   v. Post-natal history
2. To find out intrauterine growth retardation.
3. To follow Apgar score for properly assessing the newborn.
4. Thorough examination of the baby.
5. Recording anthropometric measurements of the newborn.

Neonatal History Taking

a. *Antenatal history:* Should include obstetric history, maternal illness during or before pregnancy, maternal drug intake during pregnancy, history of diabetes, oligo or polyhydramnios, intranatal and post-natal history, to know notable intrapartum procedures like breech presentation or forceps delivery.

   Extremes of age during first pregnancy have some adverse effects. Maternal ages below 18 years and above 35 years are often associated with (i) Pre-term babies, (ii) Down syndrome and (iii) Chromosomal anomalies.

   Effects of some of the medicines consumed by the mother during early part of pregnancy have been emphasised for a long-time, specially their deleterious effects on limb formation. Malformations have been noted with the ingestion of phenytoin sodium, antimalarials and sodium valproate, the last named drug is suggestive of producing spina bifida.

   Diabetic mothers may have babies with vertebral anomalies, femoral hypoplasia and caudal regression syndrome.

   Increased or decreased quantity of amniotic fluid may produce some defects in the babies like foetal limb defects and club foot from oligohydramnios; Down syndrome, Klippel Feil syndrome, acondroplasia, multiple congenital anomalies syndromes and anencephaly from polyhydramnios.

   Breech presentation—Many of the neonatal problems are caused by unusual presentation of the baby at birth. About 3 per cent of babies, who are born by breech presentation have some foetal and maternal factors as the cause. Orthopaedic problems like congenital dislocation of hip, myotonic dystrophy, Down syndrome, hydrocephalus are some of the important foetal factors, whereas oligo or polyhydramnios, uterine abnormalities, abnormal placental implantation, twin pregnancy, low birth weight of babies are some of the maternal factors found in breech presentation.

   The effects of breech on new born causing orthopaedic problems are minor ones like haematoma over thighs, soft tissue injuries and injuries to sternomastoid to major problems like cranial injury, Erb's or Klumpke's palsy, fracture of long bones, spinal cord injury, congenital talipes equinovarus, birth asphyxia and many others.

b. In searching for natal, neonatal, post-natal and family history the object will be to find out any deviation from the normal. In obtaining family history, the most important point is pedigree study, which may indicate a genetic disorder. An elderly primae may have a risk of delivering a baby with Down syndrome, as an old father points to achondroplasia or Marfan syndrome. It is very important to search for a number of siblings and deaths among siblings, abortions, intrauterine deaths, familial illness like diabetes or infectious diseases like tuberculosis and parental consanguinity as a primary offender before going for a detailed pedigree study in some relevant cases, where a genetic problem is found in the family tree.

To Find Any Intrauterine Growth Retardation

When the birth weight is less than the 10th percentile for that particular gestational age, it is due to intrauterine growth retardation and the babies born may show symmetrical retardation causing hypoplastic babies with diminished head size, shorter length and height but fairly adequate subcutaneous fat, having increased risk of congenital anomalies. On the contrary an asymmetrically retarded growth causes hypotrophic baby presenting with disproportionately reduced size with a relatively large sized head and remarkably reduced subcutaneous fat having post-natal problems of asphyxia, hypoglycaemia, malnutrition and massive pulmonary haemorrhage.

To Follow Apgar Score for Properly Assessing the Newborn

Virginia Apgar[1] in 1953 used this score to systematically assess birth asphyxia. She graded five clinical features at one minute of birth of the baby with scoring from 0 to 2. Recently the assessment is done upto 20 minutes at intervals of 5 minutes. The parameters taken are heart rate, respiratory effort, muscle tone, response to catheter in the nostril, and colour of the skin. False positive results are possible in cases of congenital myopathy or congenital neuropathy or acute cerebral trauma or spinal cord trauma with no foetal asphyxia and low Apgar. A total score of 10 Apgar indicates best possible condition of the infant. A score of 0 to 3 points towards immediate resuscitation of the infant.

Thorough Examination of the Baby

Orthopaedic examinations are not too many. But while doing so, any other obvious deformity like cleft lip or palate is noted and written in the history sheet.

There are some important points followed while examining newborns:
 i. The examination is done one hour after feeding
 ii. The examination should be done gently, methodically and in the presence of the mother
 iii. Those examinations which require quietness of the child are to be done first (e.g. auscultation of heart and palpation of abdomen).

The orthopaedic surgeons are usually asked by paediatricians to see a newborn after common life-threatening congenital anomalies like tracheo-oesophageal fistula, diaphragmatic hernia, ductal dependent congenital heart disease, along with others like retarded mental development and growth, genital hypoplasia, ear anomalies, neural tube defects like meningocele and encephalocele, renal agenesis with associated urinary and pulmonary problems, obvious umbilical, gastric and intestinal problems have been diagnosed by paediatric general surgeon.

Recognition of birth trauma is done carefully and systematically starting from head and neck for the presence of cephalhaematoma, catput succedaneum, skull fractures, sternomastoid tumour, mandibular fracture, brachial plexus injury, clavicle, humerus or femur fractures, presence of any petechiae or bruise, and for any visceral injury in case of severe trauma.

Anthropometric Measurements in the Newborn

Anthropometric measurements in the newborn are done as follows:
 i. Birth weight—weight recorded within one hour of birth
 ii. Length from crown to heel preferably with the help of an infantometer
 iii. Head circumference
 iv. Mid arm circumference.

In the second examination, which should be done within 24 hours of birth, and the baby having been fed one hour before the examination, a paediatric orthopaedic surgeon has to find out neuromuscular maturity by noting posture—of universal flexion, lack or excess of it; hypertonicity shows excessive flexion and hypotonicity showing lack of it. Some of the important reflexes are tested then.

Moro's reflex is tested by raising the head of supine infant and allowing it to drop by 10° on to the examiner's supporting hand or alternatively by holding the baby at an angle of 45° from the cot and then suddenly let the head fall back slightly into the palm. This reflex is not well-demonstrated in premature babies. Positive reflex shows opening of hands, extreme abduction of arms and hyperextension of spine, followed by anterior flexion and adduction of arm are shown in babies born at or after 32 weeks. Asymmetrical Moro's reflex is found in Erb's palsy, fracture clavicle or humerus and in hemiplegia.

Asymmetric tonic neck reflex: This simple test is done by rotation of the head to one side and maintaining upto the count of five and doing the same to the opposite side. A position reflex with extension of the upper limb on the side to which face is rotated with flexion of the arm on the side of the occiput having less similar participation of the lower limbs are present from 35 weeks onwards. Exaggerated reflex is a sign of cerebral injury.[2] The above two reflexes disappear at 4 to 6 months of age of the baby but may persist in cerebral palsy.

Search should then be made for Congenital Malformations

The malformations may occur in minor or major forms. Abnormalities in minor form of orthopaedic interest are comptodactyly of fifth fingers, Potter's thumb, syndactyly of second and third toes, short fourth metatarsals, infantile bow leg, spooned nails.

Major malformations of common occurrence are musculoskeletal defects like club coot, arthrogryposis, Down syndrome, limb reduction defects, CNS defects like anencephaly, spina bifida, encepalocele, hydrocephaly and microcephaly.

Defects like congenital dislocation of hip or knee, radial club hand, amniotic bands should also be looked for. Proper clinical examinations are done, if any condition is found.

Final Examination of the Baby at the Time of Discharge from the Hospital

This examination will confirm the presence of any abnormality in the baby or detect any, which has been missed in the first examination. The treatment, if not advised before, should be given and the follow-up intervals are informed. CNS abnormalities, if any, are confirmed by re-examination.

REFERENCES

1. Apgar V. A proposal for new method for evaluation of the newborn infant. Anesth. Analg 1953;32: 260.
2. Kulkarni ML. Manual of Neonatology. Jaypee Brothers Medical Publishers (P) Ltd. New Delhi, 72.

Chapter 4

Importance of Genetics in Neonatal Orthopaedic Diseases

> **Keywords:** Different genetic causes of neonatal orthopaedic disease–gene defects–single or multiple or chromosomal type of inheritance and their character.

Many of the neonatal orthopaedic diseases have a genetic background. Genetic problems lead to foetal loss or a deformed baby with or without mental retardation. Isolation of genes by pedigree and chromosome studies, by various foetal investigations, as has been mentioned in the previous chapter, or by genome studies, which will be possible in near future will help in proper genetic counselling.

INCIDENCE OF GENETIC DISORDERS AMONG NEONATES

According to Verma[1] about 2 per cent of newborn babies in India have a major congenital anomaly. Where neural tube defects are of frequent occurrence in North India, musculoskeletal defects are common in other parts of India. The incidence of chromosomal disorders among newborns is about 1 in 200 of which half will involve autosomes and half sex chromosomes.

ABNORMALITY OF GENES CAUSING GENETIC DISORDERS

There is a large number of neonatal orthopaedic conditions which may arise from abnormalities in the genes.

The basics of a gene arranged along the length of a chromosome is deoxyribonucleic acid (DNA). The chemical structure of DNA is a double strand twisted in the form of a helix and the vertical arms of this spiral structure are constituted by alternate phosphate-sugar-phosphate molecules. The sugars are linked to each other by the bases-adenine or guanine (the purines) and cytosine or thymine (the pyrimidines). Adenine always pairs with thymine and guanine pairs with cytosine. The genetic information is carried in the base fraction.

Genetic disorders may arise from abnormality in:
 a. *A single gene*: Resulting in a relatively uncommon disorder, which is of autosomal recessive or dominant inheritance. The phenotypes segregate within families and are not very common in occurrence.
 b. *Multiple genes*: Causing most of the common congenital malformations like club foot and spina bifida. Here, the multiple genetic defect is associated with environmental abnormality and hence is a multifactorial inheritance.
 c. *Chromosomes*: There may be absence or deficiency of a whole chromosome or a segment of it. The disorders produced are quite common but less than those due to multifactorial inheritance.

The pedigree pattern of genetic inheritance depends upon the responsible gene located on an autosome or sex chromosome as autosomal dominant or recessive or X-lined dominant or recessive.

INHERITED NEONATAL ORTHOPAEDIC CONDITIONS

The inheritance of common hereditary neonatal orthopaedic conditions are given below:
1. *Autosomal dominant*: For example, achondroplasia, cleidocranial dysplasia, Kniest syndrome, limb defect (polydactyly, syndactyly, brachydactyly), Osteogenesis imperfecta (type I and IV), spondyloepiphyseal dysplasia congenita.
2. *Autosomal recessive*: For example, achondrogenesis, chondrodysplasia punctata, diastrophic dwarfism, Jeune's disease, thanatophoric dwarfism, metatropic dwarfism, osteogenesis imperfecta (type II and III).
3. *X-linked*
4. *Multifactorial (sporadic)*: For example, CDH, CTEV.
5. *Variable uncertain*: For example, chondrodysplasia punctata, thanatophoric dwarfism.
6. *Environmental*: For example, amniotic bands.

Types of Inheritance and their Characteristics

The human zygote which receives one set of 22 pairs of autosomes from each of the parents receive also X and Y sex chromosomes one each from each of the parents who have XY (the father) and XX (the mother) chromosomes and they become either a male or a female baby. Incidentally, the chromosomes are paired structures located in the nuclei of cells.

Like chromosomes, the genes located on chromosomes are in pairs and each of the pair is known as alleles. If the pairs are different the phenotypes or the individual is heterozygous and when the pairs are same, the person is homozygous.

Autosomal Dominant Inheritance

A mutant gene which produces a permanent change, i.e. a phenotypic effect even when present in a single dose is considered as dominant gene. The progeny of a person of autosomal dominant trait will have a 50 per cent chance of carrying the mutant gene. So, the pedigree characteristics will be (a) half the children of an affected parent will be affected, irrespective of sex; (b) unaffected individuals do not transmit the trait; (c) there is a male to male transmission.

Most patients with such inheritance are heterozygous. Homozygous state, when present produces a lethal effect, e.g. lethal achondroplasia.

Autosomal Recessive Inheritance

An autosomal recessive gene produces its effect when it is homozygous in character, or in other words both parents contribute the abnormal gene to the affected child. If the recessive trait is rare, related individuals are more likely to be heterozygous for the same mutant gene. On an average one-fourth of the children of heterozygous parents are affected, half the children are carrier and one-fourth are normal.

X-linked Recessive Inheritance

Males receive one X-chromosome from the mother and one Y chromosome from the father; but the females receive one X-chromosome from both the parents. In case of heterozygous females, their sons have equal chance of inheriting the X-chromosome carrying the mutant gene.

So, the disorder almost always appears in males; affected males transmit the gene to all their daughters and not to their sons; so the daughters become carriers. Each son of a carrier female has had 50 per cent risk of being affected. The examples of such conditions are haemophilia A and B, Duchenne and Becker muscular dystrophy and Hunter syndrome.

X-linked Dominant Inheritance

The effect of mutant genes in this type of inheritance is on both females and males. One example is hypophosphatemic (vitamin D resistant) rickets.

In an affected female half of her sons and daughters will be affected, whereas in an affected male none of the sons but all the daughters will be affected. So, the female preponderance, though will be twice more than the males in a given pedigree, the disease is milder in the females. There is no male to male transmission.

From the above description of mode of inheritance and its effect, it is clear that the morphogenesis of the body depends upon autosomes whereas the development of gonads and external genitalia depends upon sex chromosomes. The most common chromosomal abnormality, e.g. trisomy G or Down syndrome involve the smallest chromosome. In the karyotyping larger chromosomal abnormalities are found only in aborted foetus, because those are incompatible with life. Abnormalities of sex chromosomes like XXY or XO will cause sterility but will not produce any change in other parts of the body except in Turner syndrome where we get somatic abnormalities.

CAUSE OF GENETIC DISORDERS

Genetic disorders are caused by some changes in the DNA induced by advanced maternal or paternal age at conception, consanguinity, ionising radiation, some of the viruses and chemicals.

Advanced maternal age at conception—will cause chromosomal abnormality like non-disjunction in the gonadal cells. In the meiotic stage of cell division half of total 46 chromosomes from gonadal cells will go into each of the two daughter cells. Due to non-disjunction one daughter cell inherits 24 chromosomes and the other 22 chromosomes. The zygote formed by the participation of cell containing 24 chromosomes will have 47 chromosomes instead of normal 46. Examples are Trisomy 21, 18, 13, XXY, XXX and XYY. An exception is Turner syndrome (XO), possibly arising as a postzygotic event.

Advanced paternal age at conception—The offsprings of such parent had single gene mutations with autosomal dominant trait. Examples are achondroplasia, Apert syndrome, Marfan syndrome.

Consanguinity—In a consanguinous marriage, the offspring will have a marginal chance of suffering from genetic disorder, if any member of the parental family suffers from autsomal recessive disease.

Ionising radiation: Radiation to gonads may produce genetic abnormality in the offspring. This may be environmental or occupational.

Viruses—The viral disease of the mother while carrying produces diseases like cerebral palsy. This is possibly due to DNA changes in the foetus.

Chemicals—Whether chemicals in the environment produce genetic disease is not proved yet. But can we correlate the increased use to chemicals in agricultural production and food processing with an increasing incidence of genetic disease.

REFERENCE

1. Verma IC. Clinical genetics: Udani PM (Ed): Text Book of Pediatrics, 1st edn. Jaypee Brothers Medical Publishers (P) Ltd: New Delhi 1998;3: 2392-408.

Chapter 5

Congenital Malformations

Keywords: Congential malformations – etiology – screening in pregnancy at different weeks to detect various anomalies – prevention of some malformations.

CONGENITAL MALFORMATIONS

A defect in the anatomical structure of the newborn baby including the viscera within is termed as congenital malformation. Sometimes, it has got a serious effect on the health and cosmetic function and survival of the newborn, known as congenital malformation major, whereas the minor variety is free from the above effects.

When the congenital anomalies are multiple and their pathology and genetic background are similar, these form a malformation syndrome. The morphologic character of the malformation depends upon its cause. Sometimes the abnormal form, shape or position of a part of the body is caused by mechanical forces, i.e. deformation, e.g. talipes equinovarus caused by foetal constraint or due to a breakdown or interference of a normal developmental process known as disruption, e.g. amniotic bands or from abnormal organization of cells in the tissues called dysplasia. Sometimes, a known prior anomaly or

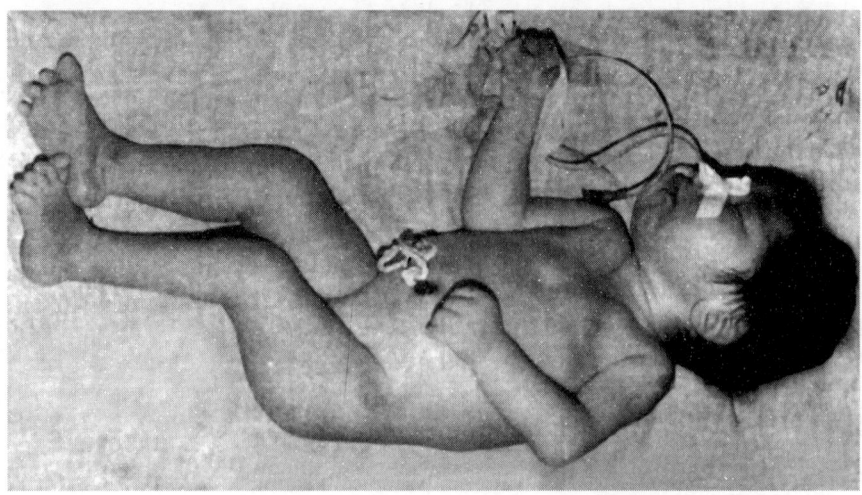

Fig. 5.1: Pierre Robin syndrome with micrognathia and cyanosis evident in the feet

Congenital Malformations

mechanical factor leads to a sequence of multiple anomalies like Pierre Robin syndrome (Fig. 5.1) or Potter syndrome.

Vertebral anomaly, anal atresia, tracheo-oesophageal fistula, radial and or renal dysplasia (VATER) or charge (coloboma, heart defect, atresia choanae, retarded growth, genital abnormality, ear anomaly) are association of some anomalies taking place as non-random occurrence in two or more individuals and not happening as a syndrome or sequence.

About three per cent of newborn children show major malformations. Only orthopaedic conditions will be described here.

Etiology

1. Single gene (4.1%)
   Autosomal dominant, e.g. achondroplasia
2. Polygenic, e.g. CTEV
   Neural tube defects.
3. Chromosomal abnormality, e.g. Down syndrome (trisomy 21) 10.1%
4. Teratogenic, e.g. Due to thalidomide-phocomelia
   Due to valporate-spina bifida, limb defects like radial ray reduction defects.
   Due to excessive alcohol intake by the mother during pregnancy—foetal alcohol syndrome.
   Due to tetracycline-enamel hypoplasia and yellow pigmentation of the teeth.
   Due to antimetabolites like aminopterin or amethopterin-hydrocephalus, craniosynostosis, shortened limbs, absent digits and mental deficiency.
   Due to anticonvalsants: Diphenhydantoin mental deficiency, microcephaly, craniofacial anomalies and nail hypoplasia.
   Due to hormones: Stilboesterol-carcinoma of vagina in female foetus and genitourinary anomaly in male foetus. Androgens and synthetic progestogens—Masculanisation of female foetus. The hormone given to the mother between 8 to 13 weeks of gestation may lead to anomalies of external genitalia and given after this period will cause cliteromegaly. Oral contraceptives—possibly heart defects, oesophageal anomalies and limb reductions.
   Radiation: In early part of gestation may cause structural defects whereas in later part of gestation radiation may lead to malformations like microcephaly.
5. Nutritional: For example, vitamin A toxicity
   Folate deficiency
6. Maternal infections: S (Syphilis) T (Toxoplasmosis) A (Australia antigen) R (Rubella) C (Cytomegalovirus) and H (Herpes) making the acronym STARCH, can affect the foetus.
   Syphilis, hepatitis due to Australia antigen and herpes infection may lead to septicemia in the foetus. Rubella, toxoplasmosis and cytomegalo virus cause mental retardation and microcephaly.
7. Maternal age: Elderly mothers giving birth to Down syndrome
8. Paternal age: Elderly fathers will give rise to achondroplastic babies.
9. Maternal condition: Like insulin dependent diabetes mellitus will cause sacral agenesis, femoral hypoplasia, microcephaly, anencephaly, spina bifida, hemivertebra and the like.
10. Multifactorial inheritance: Several minor abnormal genes and environmental factors may cause defects like celft lip and palate, hypospadias, CDH and cardiac abnormalities.
11. Vascular insufficiency: Placental thrombi may cause absence of distal limb structures.[1] Anomalies of the radial artery has been the causative factor for radial aplasia.[2] Poland syndrome is found to be due to vascular deficiency in the proximal subclavian artery, developed prior to 6th week of intrauterine period. The cause of Möbius syndrome and Klippel-Feil syndrome is attributed to vascular defect.[3]
12. Maternal Rh isoimmunisation: The condition of foetus inheriting antigen from the father, which is lacking in the mother's blood, is liable to produce maternal Rh isoimmunisation causing interference to normal foetal development.

Screening in Pregnancy for Congenital Malformations

1. The earliest screening done is between 9 to 12 weeks and that is chorionic villous biopsy (transcervical and transabdominal) for chromosomal anomalies. For inborn errors of metabolism, the biopsy is done between 12 to 20 weeks.
2. There are a number of investigations done at 12 weeks:
    i. Transvaginal ultrasonography for structural defects, anencephaly, limb defects.
    ii. Foetal cells detection in maternal circulation for foetal sex and DNA studies.
3. Between 12 to 14 weeks, the investigations done are:
   Early amniocentesis is done for chromosomal anomalies and neural tube defects. Routine amniocentesis is done a little later between 14 to 16 weeks. The earliest magnetic resonance imaging done for structural anomalies is between 12 to 16 weeks.
4. At 14 weeks, a number of investigations are done:
    i. Alpha foetoprotein (AFP) levels in maternal circulation for neural tube defects (level increased) and in Down syndrome (level decreased).
    ii. Maternal human chorionic gonadotrophin: Increased in Down syndrome.
    iii. Maternal unconjugated oestriol in serum is studied for Down syndrome when the value is decreased.
5. Between 16 and 22 weeks, a number of investigations are done:
    i. Earliest which can be done is transabdominal ultrasonography.
    ii. Foetoscopy is done between 17 and 20 weeks for foetal blood sampling for haemophilia.
    iii. Cordocentesis is done at 18 weeks for foetal blood sampling for various tests like chromosomal, biochemical, enzyme and DNA study.
    iv. Foetal echocardiography is done at 20 weeks for the detection of syndromes associated with congenital heart disease.
6. X-ray studies are done in second and third trimesters to detect skeletal dysplasias and multiple pregnancies.

Prevention of Some of the Congenital Malformations

The occurrence of neural tube defects can be prevented in three-fourth of cases by the application of 4 mgm of folic acid per day, to be started 2 months before the conception and to be continued for three months after the conception, as suggested by Vitamin study group of Medical Research Council of Great Britain.

To prevent many malformations in diabetic mothers pre-conceptional control of blood sugar level to within normal level, specially the glycosylated haemoglobin level, is necessary.

REFERENCES

1. Hoyme HE, Jones KL, Van Allen MI, et al. Vascular pathogenesis of transverse limb reduction defects. J Pediatr 1982;101:839-843.
2. Van Allen MI, Hoyme HE, Jones KL. Vascular pathogenesis of limb defects: 1. Radial artery anatomy in radial aplasia. J Pediatr 1982;101: 832-38.
3. Bouwes Bavinck JN, Weaver DD. Subclavian artery supply disruption sequence: Hopothesis of vascular etiology for Poland, Klippel-Feil and Moebius anomalies. Am J Med Gent 1986;23:903-18.

Chapter 6

General Abnormalities of Skeletal Development, Evident at Birth

Keywords: Skeletal dysplasia presenting at birth including dwarfism present in birth.

There is a plethora of diseases due to general abnormalities of skeletal development presenting at birth. Classification of such a huge list of diseases was an enormous task. Fairbank[1] in 1951 was the first to classify these defects, which he published as an atlas. His atlas was replenished with further addition of newer defects by Wynne-Davies.[2] I shall follow the Paris Nomenclature for constitution disorders of bone as the basis for the classification of dysplasias presenting at birth[3] (Table 6.1).

DWARFISM PRESENTING AT BIRTH

The list of disorders causing dwarfism present at birth (DPB) is given in a tabular form (Table 6.2).

The diseases listed in Table 6.2 and presenting as dwarfs at birth are diagnosed by the appearance of head, limbs, spine and pelvis. Most of them are autosomal recessive in origin except achondroplasia, Apert syndrome and Kniest disease, which are autosomal dominant. The dwarfism may be general and proportionate and is due to endocrine, chromosomal or metabolic causes or disproportionate dwarfing with shorter limbs or shorter trunk or may be due to low birth weight.

SIGNS OF DWARFISM AT BIRTH IN DIFFERENT DISEASES

Conradi's Disease or Chondrodysplasia Punctata

The condition affecting equally in both sexes is due to cartilaginous dysplasia with abnormal epiphyseal centres. The presence of stippled epiphyses at birth is pathognomonic. The head of the baby shows saddle nose, sloping eyes and bilateral cataract. The neck and trunk are short.

The limbs show disproportionate shortening of proximal parts of limbs with a symmetrically bowed humeri and femora, enlarged joints and flexion contractures of hips and knees. There may be dislocation of hips. Feet show marked planovalgus. There is shortening of long bones as the child grows.

The shortening of trunk and neck often associated with scoliosis is due to vertebral anomalies. The baby suffers from mental retardation and optic atrophy. The occasional associated abnormalities are various types of skin disorders, congenital heart disease, tracheo-oesophageal fistula, imperforate anus.[2]

Radiographic features include extra-cartilaginous calcification often involving vertebral column, besides stippling of the epiphyses. Separate centres of ossification for the vertebral bodies, one for the anterior part and one for the posterior part of the body may be present. There is metaphyseal cupping and splaying of the long bones. Craniostenosis is often present.

Table 6.1: General abnormalities of skeletal development, evident at birth

I.	Due to cartilaginous dysplasias:		
	A.	Cartilaginous dysplasis with abnormal epiphyseal centres chondrodysplasia punctata (Conradi disease) with dwarfism present at birth (DPB).	
	B.	Cartilaginous dysplasias with proliferation of growth-plate chondroblasts:	
		i.	Enchondromatosis (dyschondroplasia, Ollier's disease)
		ii.	Osteochondromatosis (diaphyseal aclasis, hereditary multiple exostoses).
	C.	Cartilaginous dysplasias with abnormal maturation of growth-plate chondroblasts:	
		i.	Achondroplasia (DPB)
		ii.	Metatropic dysplasia (DPB)
		iii.	Kniest disease (DPB)
		iv.	Thanatophoric dwarfism (DPB)
		v.	Achondrogenesis (DPB)
	D.	Spondylo-epiphyseal dysplasias:	
		i.	Spondylo-epiphyseal dysplasia congenita (DPB)
		ii.	Pseudochondroplasia
II.	Bone dysplasias due to abnormal bone growth		
	i.	Osteogenesis imperfecta congenita (DPB)	
	ii.	Osteopetrosis congenita (DPB)	
	iii.	Diaphyseal dysplasia	
	iv.	Osteodysplasty (Melnick-Needle syndrome) (Autosomal recessive form is lethal in the perinatal period)	
	v.	Melorheostosis	
	vi.	Neurofibromatosis with congenital localised gigantism	
	vii.	Cleidocranial dysplasia	
	viii.	Chondro-ectodermal dysplasia (Ellis-van Creveld syndrome) (DPB)	
	ix.	Asphyxiating thoracic dysplasia (Jeune's disease) (DPB)	
	x.	Campomelic dysplasia	
	xi.	Osteo-onycho dysplasia (Nail-patella syndrome)	
	xii.	Hereditary progressive arthro-ophthalmopathy (Sticklar's syndrome)	
III.	Mesomelic dysplasias		
	i.	Foetal face syndrome (DPB)	
IV.	Head and upper limb syndromes		
	i.	Acrocephalosyndactyly (Apert syndrome (DPB)	
	ii.	Acrocephalosyndactyly (Carpenter syndrome)	with polydactyly and syndactyly
	iii.	Mandibulofacial dystosis (Treacher-Collins syndrome)	

Contd...

General Abnormalities of Skeletal Development, Evident at Birth

Contd...

	iv.	Mandibular hypoplasia (Pierre Robin syndrome)
	v.	Oculo-mandibulo-facial syndrome (Hallermann-Streiff syndrome)
	vi.	Oculo-dento-osseous dysplasia
	vii.	Oro-facial-digital syndrome (Papillon-Leage syndrome)
	viii.	Cranio-carpo-tarsal syndrome (Freeman-Sheldom syndrome; Whistling face syndrome)
	ix.	Rubinstein-Taybi syndrome
	x.	Pancytopenia-dysmeila syndrome (Fanconi's anaemia)
V.	Pterygium syndromes	
	i.	Multiple pterygium syndrome (Escobar syndrome)
	ii.	Cornelia de Lange syndrome (DPB)
	iii.	Foetal dwarfism (DPB)
	iv.	Foetal alcohol syndrome
VI.	Dwarfism presenting at birth (DPB) The problem lies with identifying these defects in the neonatal period. A major group presents as dwarfs, where the dwarfism is evident at birth. The presenting defect may be due to cartilaginous dysplasias, due to abnormal bone growth, may present as mesomelic dysplasias, head and upper limb syndrome, or pterygium syndrome.	

Table 6.2: Dwarfism presenting at birth	
A.	Due to cartilaginous dysplasias with abnormal epiphyseal centres, e.g. conradi disease or chondrodysplasia punctata.
B.	Due to cartilaginous dysplasias with abnormal maturation of growth-plate condroblasts, e.g. Achondroplasia Metatropic dysplasia Kniest disease Thanatophoric dwarfism Achondrogenesis
C.	Metaphyseal chondrodysplasia, e.g. Diastrophic dysplasia
D.	Spondylo-epiphyseal dysplasia, e.g. spondylo-epiphyseal dysplasia congenita
E.	Bone dysplasias due to abnormal bone growth. For example, Osteogenesis imperfecta congenita Osteopetrosis congenita Chondro-ectodermal dysplasia (Ellis-van Creveld syndrome) Asphyxiating thoracic dysplasia (Jeune's disease)
F.	Mesomelic dysplasias, e.g. foetal face syndrome
G.	Head and upper limb syndromes, e.g. Acrocephalosyndactyly (Apert syndrome)
H.	Pterygium syndromes, e.g. Cornelia de Lange syndrome
I.	Neonatal rickets

The gross pathologic changes are abnormalities of the enchondral bone formation with reduced vascularity and little calcification. The cause of radiographic stippling[4] is polymorphous chalky deposits of circumscribed nature.

The condition is to be differentiated from multiple epiphyseal dysplasia with multiple epiphyseal ossification centres when the stipplings in X-ray are of larger sizes.[5] In some chromosomal anomalies with pre-natal radiographic stipplings are present in long bones epiphysis and not in vertebral epiphysis.

The disease is of autosomal recessive inheritance. Some of the affections are due to parental consanguinity. The disease is quite different from the milder variety—the Conradi-Hunermann type of mostly autosomal dominant inheritance, which is not usually present at birth. The babies suffering from this condition die of respiratory infection and rarely cross the first year of life.

Lengthening of long bones on a few fortunate living babies at a later age is never successful as there is fibrous union on many occasions at the site of lengthening.

Achondroplasia

This commonest form of dwarfism is due to disturbance in the division and maturation of growth-plate chondroblasts resulting in a deficiency of chondroid and improper endochondral growth. The incidence is 1 in 26,000 live births. Although the inheritance is autosomal dominant in nature, 80 per cent of the cases are due to spontaneous mutation. The diagnosis of the condition is possible at birth from the typical features of the disease having shorter lower limbs relative to the length of the trunk, the midpoint of the body being above the umbilicus. The head is disproportionately large with a bulging forehead and a low nasal bridge. The hands are short and broad with the middle and ring fingers spread apart creating a V-shaped space in between, commonly known as a trident hand. The fingers are stubby with a particularly short middle finger.

The radiological appearance of the condition at birth is evident in the metacarpals, which are almost equal in sizes; the pelvis having a quadrilateral shaped acetabulum with flat and broad acetabular roof and the sacrum articulating low on the ilia, the sciatic notches being smaller than usual. The centre of the pelvic inlet from margin is greater than its depth giving it an appearance of a champagne glass. The changes in the spine at birth are the typical appearance of the body like a bullet, an increased lumbosacral angle, narrow caudal spinal canal with short pedicles. The skull is large with a relatively short base. The metaphyses of long bones show flare with splaying and the epiphyseal cartilage is notched or V-shaped giving a ball and socket appearance to the epiphyseometaphyseal junction (Figs 6.1 and 6.2).

Diagnosis of achondroplasia can be made prenatally—homozygous cases can be diagnosed during the second trimester and heterozygous ones in the third trimester.

Metatropic Dysplasia

This rare deformity with an incidence of 2 per million presents at birth with longer trunk relative to the lower limbs. The trunk, however, becomes shorter as the child grows to the age of 2 to 3 years, due to development of kyphoscoliosis and lumbar lordosis. The condition was first described by Maroteaux et al.[6] The transmission of heredity is autosomal recessive in character. Difficulty in the establishment of normal respiration at birth because of restricted chest mobility arouses suspicion of the condition. The short limbs with enlarged knobly joints without any craniofacial changes differentiate the condition from achondroplasia. A long and narrow thorax and a triangular fold of skin overlying the tip of the coccyx characterise the disorder.

The characteristic radiological changes at birth are the extremely short long bones having constricted diaphysis and expanded ends with delayed appearances of ossification centres. Although the digits are clinically long, show radiologically short phalanges. The pelvis shows enlarged acetabulum with horizontal roofs and characteristic supra-acetabular notch, broad iliac crests with smaller greater sciatic notches and short pubic bones. The spine at birth shows platyspondyly amounting to thinning

General Abnormalities of Skeletal Development, Evident at Birth

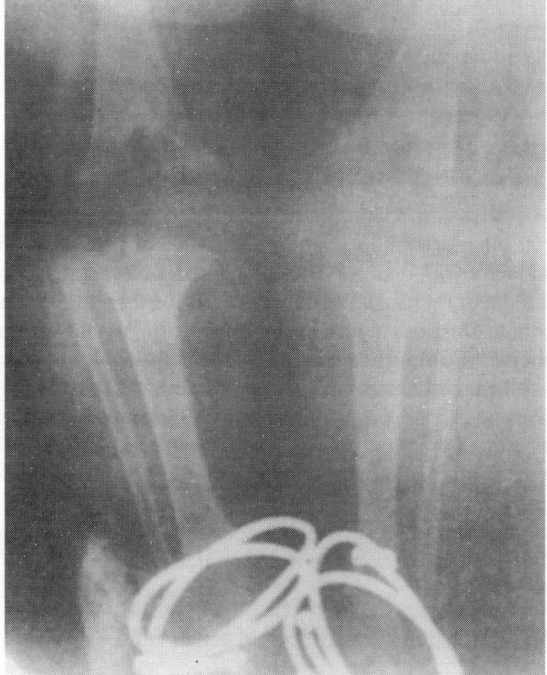

Fig. 6.1: Splaying of the metaphyses of the bones around the knees with V-shaped epiphyseal plates of lower femora and relatively increased length of the fibulas in achondroplasia

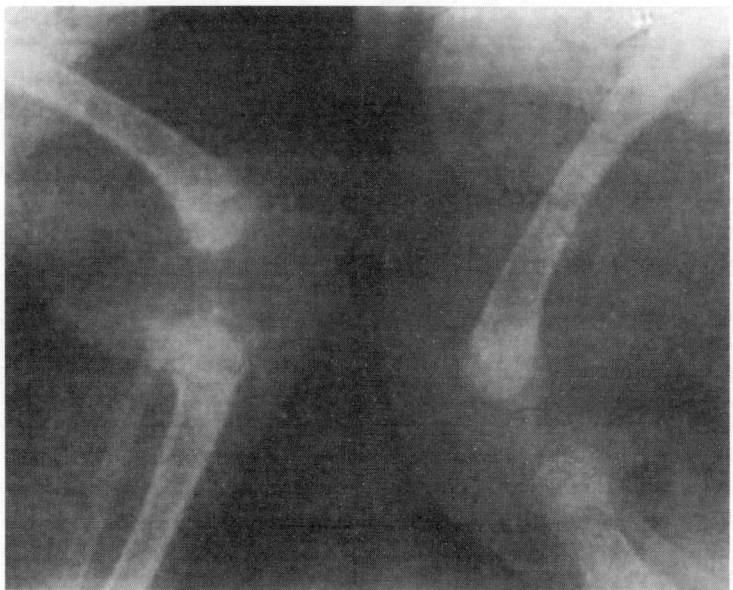

Fig. 6.2: Lateral view of the same patient mentioned in Figure 6.1

of the vertebral bodies with narrowing of the interpedicular distance in the lumbar spine from above downwards. Sometimes atlanto-axial instability is detected at birth, when after due care to the condition at early age atlanto-axial or occipito-cervical fusion is done at a later age.

Kniest Disease

Like metatropic dysplasia, this is also a short-trunk dwarfism of disproportionate character with Kyphoscoliosis, typical facies and limited joint movement but of autosomal dominant inheritance.

The physical finding at birth are stiffness and deformities of joints, long and knobly fingers with limited flexion, typical flat facies with hypertelorism, having depressed nasal bridge, prominent myopic eyes amounting to detachment of retina, cleft palate and hearing loss but with normal intelligence.

The condition is difficult to diagnose at birth but the suspicion arises later on because of delayed and painful walking due to joint pain. Radiological features[7] of platyspondyly with vertebral clefts, hypoplastic pelvic bones with dumb-bell shaped femora are evident at birth. The iliac bones are broad with narrow wine-glass pelvic inlet, the acetabula being irregular with honeycomb appearance. Later on the hands show delayed epiphyseal ossification and osteopenia.

The condition is due to an abnormality of cartilage proteoglycan metabolism evident at increased urinary excretion of keratosulphate.

Prevention of flexion contracture of hips and knees by passive joint movements, exercises and splintage is the initial treatment to be adopted in the neonatal period.

Thantophoric Dwarfism

This autosomal recessive condition is not compatible with life as most of the babies die in infancy of respiratory inadequacy. The dwarfism is characterised by a large head, narrow thorax, extremely short limbs having telephone receiver like femora and normal length of trunk. Radiologically, the vertebral bodies are flat, the ribs are short, the pelvis presents features of acondroplasia and the long bones are bent with flared metaphyses.

Achondrogenesis

A baby born with quite a large head, normal trunk and severely shortened limb should arise suspicion of achondrogenesis. Radiographs of spine and pelvis do not show the spine, sacrum, pubis and ischium clearly because of poor mineralisation. The condition is autosomal recessive in nature and most of them are born dead or die in infancy.

Diastrophic Dysplasia

This defect is due to abnormal collagen organisation of cartilage and the term is derived from the Greek word meaning crooked or twisted. The baby with this deformity at birth shows shortening of the distal segments more than the proximal ones, limited joint movements talipes equinovarus and deformity of thumb in abduction and extension. Often the middle finger is short with a gap between the ring and little on the ulnar side and the index and middle on the radial side. In the first month of life irregular swellings appear on external ears which are like blisters at the onset, gradually calcified and ultimately ossified. The face with full cheeks show flared nostrils with narrow bridge of the nose, cleft palate and hypoplastic mandible. As expected with diastrophic dysplasia the spine also becomes Kyphoscoliotic usually at around the prepubertal age. The stature thus becomes shortened with age. The inheritance is autosomal recessive and the abnormal gene is located on the distal long arm of chromosome 5. The largest series is from Finland by Poussa et al.[8]

Radiological appearance at birth shows narrowing of upper part of thorax; the spine showing flattening of vertebral bodies with Kyphosis and occasional subluxation in the cervical spine. The pelvis is normal but the hips may show subluxation. Other limb joints are often deformed and subluxated. The first metatarsals and metacarpals are often oblong in shape resulting in a varus great toe and abducted and extended thumb. The long bones show short and thick diaphysis with enlarged metaphysis.

Treatment of deformities of the feet by manipulation and plaster casts or by splints often fail because of inherent defect in the bones of the feet. Soft tissue surgery is needed in those cases. Deformities and subluxation in joints need correction by surgery. Late onset of spinal deformites are corrected by early fusion. Cervical subluxation is often associated with quadriplegia necessitating in decompression. But the prognosis is poor.

Spondyloepiphyseal Dysplasia Congenita

This disproportionate dwarfism having an incidence of 1 to 2 per million with shortened trunk due to thoracic Kyphosis with marked lumbar lordosis and absence of ossification in some of the lower limb bones, is evident at birth. Characteristic facies having hypertelorism, high arched palate and short neck in a baby with a short trunk helps in the clinical diagnosis at birth. With growth the shortening of trunk becomes more pronounced. Epiphyses of the long bones, particularly those of the proximal and distal femora and the proximal tibia are progressively involved. The epiphyses are delayed in appearance, late to ossify and show irregular growth both in the vertebrae and long bones. The vertebrae show platyspondyly and the joints of limbs become deformed specially in the hip in the form of coxa vara. Sometimes the joints are dislocated. The thorax is barrel shaped with pectus excavatum. Because of dysplasia of odontoid process there is development of atlanto-axial dislocation or subluxation. Eye changes like myopia, cataract, retinal detachment are common in adolescence. The inheritance is autosomal dominent linked to chromosome 12q.13.

Radiological changes at birth show absence of ossification of the distal femur, proximal tibia, pubic bones, tali and calcaneus. The pelvis is evident with broad ilia, femoral shafts present lateral bending and the spine shows platyspondyly and thoraco-lumbar kyphosis.

The condition is to be differentiated from Morquio's syndrome by the absence of keratan sulphate in the urine and from pseudoachondroplasia by marked changes in the limbs sometimes amounting to a windswept deformity with valgus knee and adducted hip on one side and a varus knee and abducted hip on the other.

The treatment in old children is correction of dislocation of limb joints and cervico-occipital fusion if there is dislocation or subluxation of the cervical spine.

Osteogenesis Imperfecta

This genetically heterogenous condition with a fragile skeleton has several varieties according to the severity of involvement and genetic inheritance. The severity may vary from a stillborn baby with multiple fractures to a milder variety with slight tendency to fracture.

Osteogenesis imperfecta congenita which is present at birth, often with multiple fractures, will be discussed here. Osteogenesis imperfecta tarda usually develop fracture when the child learns walking, but the condition of osteopenia and cortical thinning of bone are present in a hitherto normal radiograph.

Classification and Incidence

The condition is best described according to Sillence[9] classification which is comprehensive and thorough. He has described four types with types I and IV divided into A and B and Type II divided into A, B and C. All are autosomal dominant in inheritance except type IIC and Type III, which are autosomal recessive. The type II is osteogenesis imperfecta congenita A and the type III and IVA are congenita B as described by Shapiro.[10]

The incidence varies between 1 in 30,000 in type I and 1 in 62,000 in type II; the incidence of other two varieties is not known yet.

Etiology

Biochemical defects in the genes for collagen A1 and A2 cause this connective tissue disorder. In the congenita A and B varieties of Shapiro, i.e. Type II A, B, C and Type III and Type IVB of Sillence the collagen A1 and A2 produced is mostly structurally abnormal with molecular defect. In the Sillence Type I variety the cause is 50 per cent underproduction of normal collagen A1, i.e. a quantitative change. The defect in both the qualitative and quantitative varieties is in chromosome 7q21.

Clinical Features

Fragility of bones causing fracture is common in all the varieties; but in type I and type IV bone fragility is never severe and fractures occur later in life with a lesser incidence than in other types (Table 6.1).

The incidence and severity of deformities due to fractures is more in type II and III, i.e. in more serious type of the disease. Sometimes babies are born with birth fractures in the long bones, ribs and skull with even subdural haematoma or develop fracture without any significant trauma. One bone may fracture repeatedly, which indicates a milder form of the disease. Fracture are common to occur in the lower limbs. The multiplicity of fractures make the children fearful (Fig. 6.3). Otherwise, the suffering children are bright and intelligent.

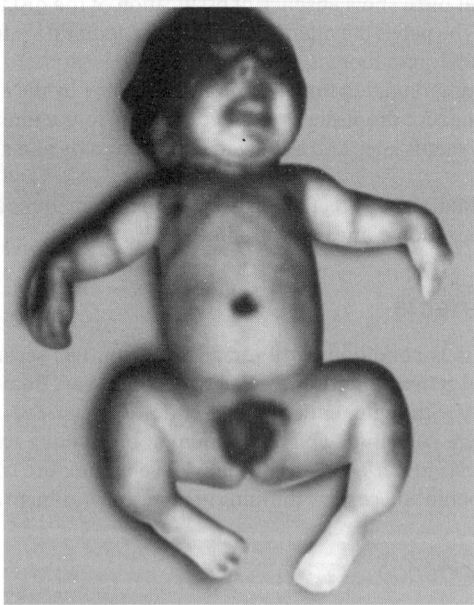

Fig. 6.3: Clinical photograph of a crying baby with multiple fractures in both upper and lower limbs in osteogenesis imperfecta

Blueness of sclera, which is due to thinness of scleral collagen, is present in type I and II. The sclera is blue at birth in type III but becomes normal in adulthood and is absolutely normal in type IV. Sometimes the sclera surrounding the cornea is white with a further ring in the periphery of sclera producing what is known as arcus juvenilis. Blue sclera is not associated with any visual impairment.

Hypermobility of joints due to laxity of ligaments is a common finding in osteogenesis imperfecta. This is again due to collagen abnormality. Pes valgus, genu recurvatum, patello femoral instability, hyperextended elbow, atlantoaxial subluxation and occasional hip and radial head dislocation are found due to laxity of ligaments.

Problems arise with teeth, starting from late eruption, brittleness, proneness to caries to abnormal teeth from deficiency of dentin. The colour of the teeth both deciduous and permanent varies between yellowish brown and translucent blue.

In adults the symptoms like Kyphoscoliosis and deafness from otosclerosis develop in about one-third of cases with osteogenesis imperfecta.

The clinical features of Type II A, B and C and Type III and Type IVA which Shapiro[10] described as congenita A and congenita B respectively are given in a tabular form[11] in Table 6.3.

Radiographic features: The X-ray findings of osteogenesis imperfecta are characteristic at birth and in the neonatal period. The long bones which are wide at diaphysis equalling metaphysis with thin cortices show multiple fractures at various stages of healing (Fig. 6.4). Some of the long bones are, therefore, angulated and some are accordion-like or crampled. The ribs are beaded with atrophy of the thoracic cage; and the skull shows practically no ossification (Fig. 6.5). The other redeeming feature is osteoporosis. The presence of wormian bones at the suture lines is characteristically present in the nonossified membranous skull bones of osteogenesis imperfecta like cleidocranial dysostosis.

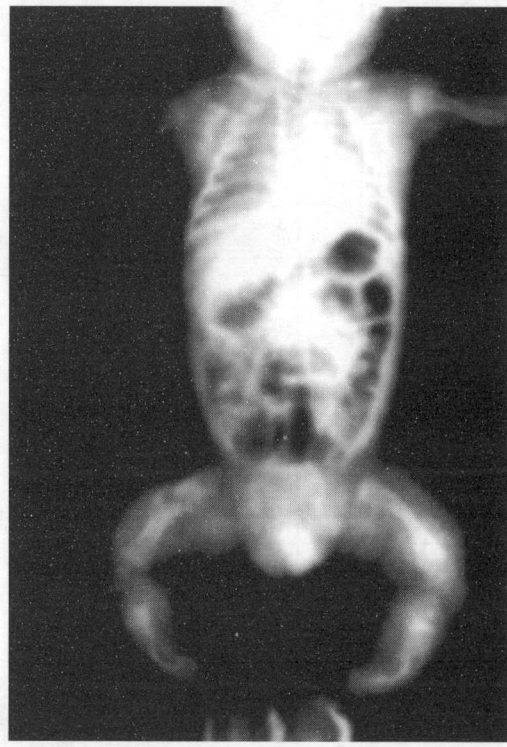

Fig. 6.4: Osteogenesis imperfecta with multiple fractures at various stages of healing

Table 6.3: Clinical features according to types of Sillence in congenita A and B

	Congenita A: Type II			Congenita B		Type IVA
	A	B	C	Type III		
Inheritance	Autosomal dominant	Autosomal dominant	Autosomal recessive	Autosomal recessive	Autosomal recessive	Autosomal dominant
Incidence	1 in 62,000	Not known	Extremely rare	Very rare		Unknown
Bone fragility	Very severe	Very severe	Very severe	Severe, numerous fractures by 2 years of age		Moderate-newborn fracture-25%
Deformity of long bones	Broad, crumpled accordion-like, specially femurs and humerus; beaded ribs	Broad, crumpled; beaded ribs; rib fractures	Thin, fractured long bones; ribs slightly beaded	Fractures at birth; severe deformities of long bones		Moderate
Hyperimobility of joints-ligamentous laxity	Unknown because of perinatal death	Unknown because of perinatal death	Unknown because of perinatal death	Marked		Moderate
Spine deformity	?	?	?	Severe kyphoscoliosis; cod fish vertebrae		Kyphoscoliosis
Skull	Wormian bones with severe demineralisation	Wormian bones with severe demineralisation	Wormian bones with severe demineralisation	Membranous bones, severe deossification; Wormian bones; occiput, facial bones fairly well ossified; triangular facies		Moderate-deossification; Wormian bones
Teeth	Unknown because of perinatal death	Unknown because of perinatal death	Unknown because of perinatal death	Dentinogenesis imperfecta		Normal
Sclerae	Blue	Blue	Blue	Blue at birth and infancy, but becomes normal later		Normal
Deafness	—	—	—	—		Deafness less severe-otosclerosis
Other	Flattened acetabuli; microscopic calcification of aorta and endocardium	Flattened acetabuli	Flattened acetabuli	'Popcorn' calcification		
Prognosis	Perinatal lethal respiratory disease	Survival possible; respiratory disease	Perinatal lethal respiratory disease	Wheelchair bound; Utmost household ambulator		
Chondro-osseous and biochemial defect	Collagen produced structurally abnormal	Collagen produced structurally abnormal	Collagen produced Structurally abnormal	Collagen produced structurally abnormal		—

General Abnormalities of Skeletal Development, Evident at Birth

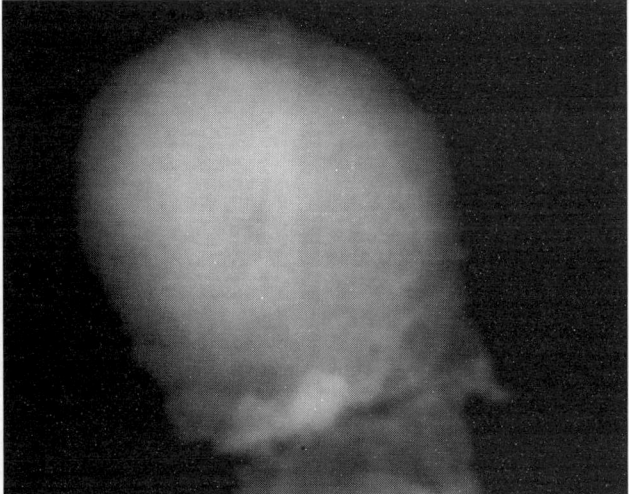

Fig. 6.5: Skull in osteogenesis imperfecta showing practically no ossification

Differential Diagnosis

Various other conditions like achondroplasia, camptomelic dwarfism or congenital hypophosphatasia with multiple fractures in the neonatal period or at birth with short limbs and enlarged head must be differentiated from osteogenesis imperfecta by radiological studies and skin biopsy for study of collagen. The conditions mimicking osteogenesis imperfecta in older children are omitted here.

Treatment

A baby born with multiple fractures in the long bones, ribs and skull needs particular care in handling the baby, maintenance of respiration in multiple rib fractures even by an anaesthesiologist and the help of a neurosurgeon is asked for in case of subdural haematoma following skull fracture.

The problem needs to be discussed with the parents, not only for the initial management of simple splintage for multiple fractures but also regarding the upbringing of the child when the need for correction of bent bones and kyphoscoliosis will arise (Figs 6.6 and 6.7). As the callus formation occurs early (Fig. 6.8) the immobilisation by splintage should be done for a short period to prevent development of osteoporosis.

The osteoporosis in this disease is real problem (Fig. 6.9) and various types of medicines tried for the condition are proved useless. Further development of fractures from osteoporosis is prevented by different types of orthosis, which again help in the locomotion of the child. The difficulty in locomotion arises from improper muscular development due to bone and joint immobilisation by various types of splints and orthosis, so develops a vicious cycle.

In a child of three years or more, the problems arising from the disease like deformity of long bones are treated surgically. Multiple osteotomies of deformed long bones, correction of alignment and holding the fragments with various types of intramedullary rods like Sofield's and telescoping IM rods of Bailey and Dubow are undertaken at around three to five years of age. The procedure also helps in the better use of orthosis.

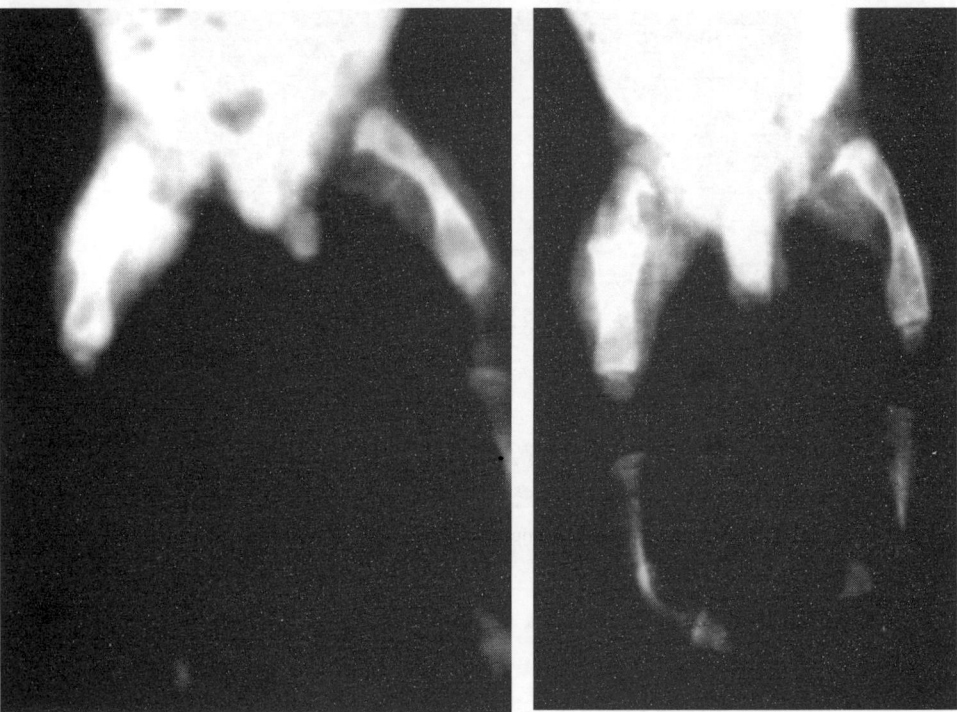

Figs 6.6 and 6.7: Bent bones in osteogenesis imperfecta showing kyphoscoliosis of tibia and fibula at two different stages

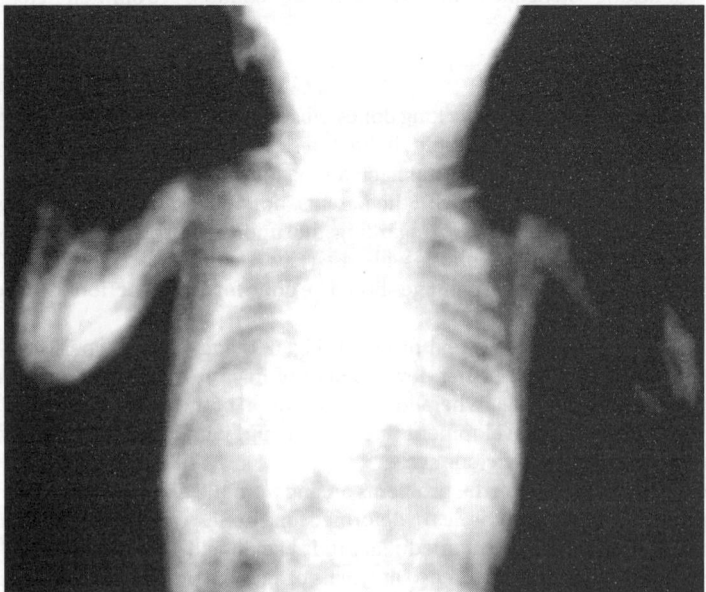

Fig. 6.8: Early callus formation in fractures in osteogenesis imperfecta

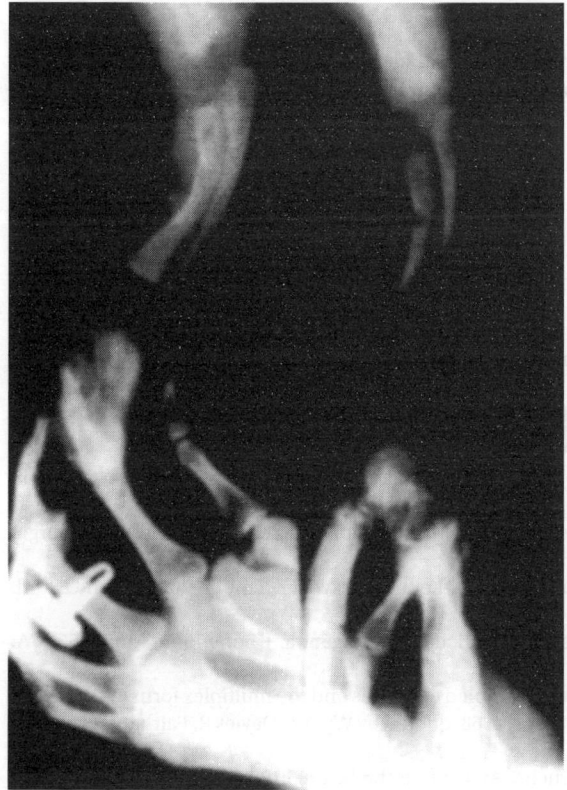

Fig. 6.9: Osteoporosis in osteogenesis imperfecta

Osteopetrosis Congenita

Report on osteopetrosis by morphological study was given by Milgram and Jasty.[12] From the ultrastructural and biochemical study of postmortem tissue from a child, who died during the neonatal period the basic defect in osteopetrosis was found to be an abnormal osteoclastic resorption of bone.[13] The death in the neonatal period proves the presence of the disease since birth.

Chondroectodermal Dysplasia (Ellis-Van Creveld Syndrome)

The dwarfism in this condition is centrifugal type, which means, the shortening is more in the lower legs and forearms than in the thighs and upper arms. The manifestations include-bowing of humeric and femora, genu valgum with subluxation or dislocation of patella, polydactyly with duplication of digits on the ulnar side, ectodermal dysplasia causing small, hypoplastic, dystrophic and spoon-shaped nails with irregular or pointed teeth, late in eruption or often present as natal teeth.[14] Dental caries is often present. The hairs are sparse. In about 60 per cent of cases congenital heart disease in the form of atrial or ventricular septal defect is present. There is often fusion between the upper lip and gums. The ribs are often short and the thoracic cage is long and narrow.

The treatment is mostly directed towards congenital heart condition. The polydactyly of hands and feet are treated by excision between one and two years of age. Genu valgum needs correction by osteotomy, when it is severe.

Asphyxiating Thoracic Dysplasia (Jeune's Disease)

Here the dwarfism is associated with long, narrow, cylindrical chest with markedly diminished antero-posterior and lateral diameter often causing asphyxiating features.

Acrocephalosyndactyly (Apert Syndrome)

It is described with craniosynostosis.

Cornelia de Lange Syndrome

Here, the dwarfism is associated with mental retardation, congenital longitudinal deficiency of the long bones, mostly postaxial that is ulnar or fibular and the patient often fails to thrive.

REFERENCES

1. Fairbank TJ. Atlas of General Affections of the Skeleton, 1st edn. Edinburgh, London, New York: Churchill Livingstone.
2. Wynne-Davies R, Fairbank TJ. Fairbank's Atlas of General Affections of the Skeleton, 2nd edn. Edinburgh, London, New York: Churchill Livingstone; 1951.p.10.
3. Sharrard WJW. Paediatric Orthopaedics and Fractures, 3rd edn. Blockwell Scientific Publication Oxford, 1:45.
4. Selakovich WG, Warren White J. Chondrodystrophia calcificans congenita. J Bone Joint Surg 1965;37A: 1271.
5. Silverman FN. Discussion on the relation between stippled epiphysis and the multiplex form of epiphysial dysplasia. Birth Defects Original Artich Series 5, Part 4, 68, quoted by Wynne-Davies R, Fairbank TJ in their Atlas, 1951;10.
6. Maroteaux, et al. Der metatropische Zwergwuchs. Arch Kinderheilk 1966;173:211, quoted by Sharrard WJM., 1993.
7. Rimoin DL, Siggers DC, Lachman RS, Siberberg R. Metatropic dwarfism, the Kniest syndrome and the pseudoachondroplastic dysplasias. Clin Orthop 1976;124:70.
8. Poussa M, Merikanto J and Associates: Spine deformities in diastrophic dysplasia. Paper read at EPOS meeting at Athens in March 1990 - quoted by Sharrard WJW 1990;1:80.
9. Sillence DO. Osteogenesis imperfecta: An expanding panorama of variants. Clin Orthop 1981;159:11.
10. Shapiro F. Consequences of an osteogenesis imperfecta diagnosis for survival and ambulation. J Pediatr Orthop 1985;5:456.
11. Tachdjian MO. Clinical Pediatric Orthopedics: The art of Diagnosis and Principles of Management. Stanford CT: Appleton and Lange.p.460.
12. Milgram JW, Jasty M. Osteopetnosis - a morphological study of twenty cases. J Bone and Joint Surg 1982;64A:912-29.
13. Shapiro Frederic, Glimcher MJ, Holtrop ME, Tashjian AK. Jr. Brickley - Parsons Diane, Kenzora JE: Human Osteopetrosis. A Histological, Ultrastructural and Biochemical Study. J Bone Joint Surg, 1980;62A:384-99.
14. Taeusch, Ballard, Avery (Eds): Schaffer and Avery's Diseases of the Newborn: 6th edn, 173, WB Saunders Co. Harcourt Brace Jovanovich, Inc: Philadelphia, London, Toronto, Montreal, Sydney, Tokyo.

Chapter 7

Disorders of Voluntary Muscles Presenting at Birth

Keywords: Congenital origin–hypotonia of skeletal muscles at birth–weakness of muscles with delayed milestones–slowly progresses – five varieties.

These disorders have some features in common like, the origin is congenital, presents with hypotonia of skeletal muscles at birth, delayed physical milestones with weakness of the muscles of the limbs. The progress of these disorders is usually slow. These diseases differ from a condition described by Walton[1] which he termed benign congenital hypotonia, where hypotonia at birth recovers completely without demonstrable pathology in the muscles.

Types of disorders of voluntary muscles presenting at birth:
  I. Genetically determined myopathy
     Congenital muscular dystrophy
     1. Type I
     2. Type II-Fukuyama variety
  II. Congenital structural myopathies
     1. Central core disease
     2. Nemaline (rod-body) myopathy
     3. Mitochondrial and storage myopathies
  III. Myotonia congenita (Thomsen's disease)
  IV. Congenital myotonic dystrophy
  V. Infantile spinal muscular atrophy

CONGENITAL MUSCULAR DYSTROPHY

There are two varieties of this genetically determined congenital myopathy of autosomal recessive type affecting both sexes equally.

The first variety or type I presents with a hypotonic baby at the time of birth with multiple joint contractures, and in some babies—a common deformity is talipes equino varus. The stiffness of the joints increases with growth. The examination reveals generalised muscle weakness mostly of the proximal part of the body more than the distal. The muscles of the face and neck are almost always affected causing difficulty in sucking and swallowing. Extra ocular muscles are however spared. The tendon reflexes are diminished or absent. The mental development is normal. The child learns walking by two years of age and reaches adulthood. The diagnosis is established by the following investigations.

Creatine phosphokinase (CPK) is normal or mildy elevated. Electromyography (EMG) shows features of myopathy. In the biopsy, there is increase of perimyseal and endomyseal connective tissue with the muscle fibres showing degeneration, regeneration and hypertrophy at places.

The treatment of this variety is by passive range-of motion exercises, and splintage from birth, and soft tissue release at a later date, where necessary. Orthotic support is given as and when required.

Type II-Fukuyama variety: In this variety of congenital myopathy described by Fukuyama[2] there is prenatal detection by the mother from less foetal movements. The sucking and crying of the newborn are weak. As the affected babies grow up half of them will develop pseudohypertrophy of the muscles with mild contractures and half will suffer from convulsion. Normal development is lacking. The baby can learn sitting up and crawling but rarely stands up. The chest of the baby is funnel shaped. The mental retardation starts from the first year of life and the child dies at about the age of ten. There can be even spontaneous abortion of such a case.

The diagnosis will be by the elevation of creatine-phosphokinase upto fifty times of normal. Blood cholesterol is also raised with myoglobinaemia. As there are mental changes, EEG shows sharp and slow waves. CT scan shows less development of gyri with dilated ventricles. EMG shows some specific changes. Cardiac muscles show focal fibrosis.

CONGENITAL STRUCTURAL MYOPATHIES

Central Core Disease

This variety of myopathy has structural change in the muscle biopsy with non-functioning central cores. This disease has had autosomal dominant inheritance.

The baby presents with hypotonia from birth, delayed physical milestones, and weakness of the muscles of the limbs. The tendon jerks are either normal or absent. The progress of the disease is slow in the majority of cases.

Nemaline (rod-body) Myopathy

This congenital myopathy is common in females with presenting features of scoliosis, pigeon chest, elongated face and high arch palate.

Mitochondrial and Storage Myopathies

This congenital myopathy with electron microscopic appearance of abnormalities of mitochondria shows a non-progressive nature with involvement of extraocular muscles and brain at times. Sometimes, myoclonus is present with lactic acidosis.

MYOTONIA CONGENITA (THOMSEN'S DISEASE)

This rare disease with myotonia is usually present at birth involving almost all the muscles of the body. The pioneering describer of this disease, Julius Thomsen himself suffered from this disease.[3]

Myotonia means failure of the muscles to relax after active contraction. The presenting symptoms after birth are peculiar strangled cry and difficulties in feeding. Cold and rest or tapping the surface of a voluntary muscle with fingertip or a percussion hammer increase myotonia. As the child grows, he feels difficulty in initiating active movements after lying down or sitting for a while. Exercise like walking relieves the myotonia. Only problem in a grown-up child is the delay in motor development on many occasions, without any definite muscle weakness or deformities.

This hereditary condition is inherited mostly by autosomal dominant transmission and rarely by recessive mode.

Diagnosis

Although creatinine phosphokinase and serum aldolase are normal the EMG shows a rapid volley of action potentials, which is diagnostic.

The condition will have to be differentiated from myotonic dystrophy, the description of which will follow.

Treatment

Myotonia usually gets better as the child becomes older. Only in rare persisting cases oral intake of quinine sulphate or procainamide is indicated.

CONGENITAL MYOTONIC DYSTROPHY

Congenital myotonic dystrophy of early onset with onset *in utero* is rarer than the late onset variety. The early variety with neonatal features occurs when the mother of the baby is also affected with the disease. The late onset variety which occurs at the end of the first decade is found when the father is affected.

The early variety, with which we are concerned, presents at birth with hypotonia, respiratory distress from weakness of the respiratory muscles and diaphragm, feeding difficulties due to difficulty in sucking from weakness of the jaw muscles, mental retardation, deformities like arthrogryposis with talipes equinovarus. The grown-up children show ptosis, dropping of the jaw, weakness of sternomastoid muscles, swallowing and speech difficulties due to palatal, pharyngeal and oesophageal involvement. Hip dislocation, hernia, undescended testes, heart defects and hydrocephalus are often found with this condition.

The early onset is easily diagnosed from reduced foetal movements reported by the mother, who herself is affected with the disease and from the presence of hydramnios in later months of pregnancy.

INFANTILE SPINAL MUSCULAR ATROPHY

This hypotonic condition of the muscles manifests at birth. This is not a myopathy but the cause is progressive degeneration of the anterior horn cells of the spinal cord and motor nuclei of 5th to 12th cranial nerves. This is a hereditary condition with autosomal dominant inheritance. The incidence of the disease is 1 in 15,000 live births. The younger the age of onset of the disease worse is the prognosis.

There are different varieties of this disease. The acute infantile type presents with hypotonia at birth and hence needs some detailing here. In the other varieties like congenital infantile type (Werdnig-Hoffman) or chronic juvenile type or Kugelberg-Welander disease, the hypotonia manifests at a later age.

The acute infantile type is very severe and extensive in nature. The degenerative process starts *in utero*. The involvement of the spinal cord begins distally and progresses proximally. So, the hypotonia is worse in the lower than in the upper limbs.

The manifestation of the acute infantile type at birth is a floppy baby due to generalised hypotonia of the voluntary muscles. There is practically very little motion in the limbs and the attitude of the baby is typical. The hips are flexed, abducted and laterally rotated and the elbows are flexed. As the child grows there is extension of the degeneration with bulbar and respiratory paralysis. Death usually occurs within one year of age.

The condition can be diagnosed by the mother from the lack of or no foetal movements in the last trimester of pregnancy.

REFERENCES

1. Walton JJ. Disorders of Voluntary Muscle, 4th edn. Edingurgh:Churchill Livingstone 1980.pp.205-37.
2. Fukuyama Y, Osawa M, Suzuki H. Congenital progressive muscular dystrophy of the Fukuyama type—clinical, genetic and pathological considerations, Brain Dev 1981;3:1.
3. Thomsen J. Tonische Kranfe in willkurlich bweglichen Muskein in Folge von erebier psychischer Disposition. Arch Psychiat Nervenkr 1876:6: 706 quoted by Tachdjian MO. Clinical Pediatric Orthopaedics The Art of Diagnosis and Principles of Management. Stanford CT: Appleton and Lange 1997;406.

Chapter 8

Can We Diagnose Cerebral Palsy in the Neonatal Period?

Keywords: Cerebral palsy – disorder of motor function – produced by some pre-natal, natal or neonatal factors – often diagnosed in the neonates from changes in the neurobehaviour as the brain is less differentiated then.

CEREBRAL PALSY

Cerebral palsy is a disorder of motor function, which develops from various pre-natal and natal factors and manifests at birth or soon after birth. The disease is of different types and presents in mild or severe form. The milder types are difficult to diagnose in the neonatal period. The pre-natal and natal history and the neurobehaviour of the baby help in the diagnosis in the neonatal period.

In the pre-natal history, the genetic and environmental causes are ascertained. Genetic aberration will cause cerebral palsy as found in Down syndrome. Environmental factors include suffering of the mother from a disease, specially a viral one like rubella or vitamin A excess, which leads to development of hydrocephalus; or alcoholism, causing microcephaly with low IQ and low birth weight. Malnutrition, anaemia, repeated convulsions, irradiation for any cause are important maternal predisposing factors.

The perinatal factors are equally important. Any birth trauma, hypoxia during delivery, hyperbilirubinemia specially excess of unconjugated bilirubin, delivery of twins, precipitate labour, forceps application causing trauma to baby or asphyxia at birth are important precipitating causes.

Post-natal infection, trauma, increased intracranial tension, vascular conditions, developing in the neonatal period, may lead to cerebral palsy.

There may not be presence of any factor described above in a particular case of cerebral palsy or if the presence of a factor is not of significance and yet the child suffers from the fateful disease, in that case an understanding of neurobehaviour is very important.

The nervous system, its pattern and problems are completely different in the neonates and in the infants. The brain is less differentiated in the neonatal period and is in the process of development. The neurological problems in this period are, therefore, assessed not from the morphological changes, but from the changes in the neurobehaviour. The biochemical changes, the changes in the properties of the membranes or any developmental defect in the neural sensorimotor circular organisation become important in the neonatal period.

The nervous system functions at two different levels. In the level of the spinal cord, it works reflexly while at the level of the brain, the cerebral cortex processes the sensory information and transform it into motor function. This is what is neurobehaviour.

The neonate suffering from cerebral palsy will behave differently from a normal neonate and the neurobehaviour will depend upon the type of insult and its effect at the stage of foetal brain development.

Protein malnutrition during pregnancy makes the proliferation and migration of brain cells a slow process. At the level of the cerebral cortex the pathology may be in the form of small loss of grey matter to a massive loss due to large cyst formation (porencephaly) causing pressure on the gyri—the result is development of microgyri. The meninges are thickened with subdural or subarachnoid haematoma formation. The results will be spasticity, mental retardation and convulsions.

Hypoxia causes oedema in the developing brain and asphyxia at birth leads to intraventricular haemorrhage if the baby is pre-mature or superficial punctate haemorrhage in a full-term baby. There are changes in the cortex and basal ganglia. All these interfere with the incorporation of aminoacids and protein synthesis and lead to learning difficulties and behaviour problems.

Hyperbilirubinemia causes kernicterus and subsequently choreoathetosis. The neurons which are pyknotic get sequential changes of chromatolysis, gliosis and demyelination. Deafness which is often seen is due to involvement of the VIII nerve nucleus.

The suspicion of diagnosis of cerebral palsy in the neonatal period will arise from feeding difficulties, vomiting, convulsions, drowsiness and jitteriness, specially in a low birth weight baby. Spontaneous involuntary movements and any unusual posture in which the baby lies are suggestive. Neurological examination when reveals predominantly flexor tone in early period with subsequently prolonged and unilateral ankle clonus, exaggerated reflexes and extensor plantar response are suggestive of cerebral palsy. The neurological findings vary with the sleepiness or wakefulness of the baby, whether he is hungry or had his food and on the body temperature. So, the neurologic examination needs to be repeated to come to a conclusion. The signs of visual, auditory or sensory involvement should also be tested. Of the common reflexes Moro, palmar and plantar grasp, the tonic neck reflex is important and tested by turning the infant's head to one side, when the ipsilateral arm extends and the contralateral one flexes with the legs following the same. A strong and persistent neck reflex, not voluntarily overcome, is suggestive of poor motor development.

Predominant dyskinesias like rapid uncoordinated voluntary movements, i.e. chorea or slow, writhing involuntary movements mostly in the distal parts of the limbs, i.e. athetosis are to be looked for. Ataxia is not very common and is associated with hypotonia and nystagmus.

EEG changes are common in cerebral palsy but EMG findings differentiate it from spinal muscular atrophy and disorders of muscle.

Chapter 9

Birth Injuries

Keywords: Birth injuries - produced by trauma during labour or delivery - due to mechanical or anoxic cause - predisposing risk factors - five different types according to body structures involved.

Trauma to a baby during labour or delivery due to some mechanical or anoxic cause, which may be avoidable or unavoidable, produces birth injury. The incidence in Western literature is 2-7 per 1,000 live births and the mortality from the condition is 5-8 per 1 lac births.[1] The incidence of birth trauma and hypoxia as a percentage of total perinatal deaths in 5,340 deliveries in Bokaro, an Indian industrial township showed perinatal mortality rate as 52.6 per 1,000 deliveries.[2]

There are some risk factors which predispose to causing birth injuries. Some of these are from maternal side, some from foetal side and some are iatrogenic.[3] The maternal causes are small stature, primiparity, pelvic abnormalities, prolonged or precipitous labour, abnormal presentation, oligohydramnios, and deep transverse arrest. From the foetal side extreme prematurity, microsomia and various anomalies may be the precipitating factors.

According to the structures of the body involved birth trauma may be of different types:
1. Head and neck injuries
2. Nerve injuries including brachial plexus injuries
3. Bone injuries
4. Intra-abdominal injuries
5. Skin and soft tissue injuries.

HEAD AND NECK INJURIES

There are various types of head and neck injuries, common among them are—cephalhaematoma, caput succedaneum, intra-cranial haemorrhage, skull fractures, sternomastoid tumour, subgaleal haematoma, mandibular fracture, and injury to the eye or ear.

Various cranial injuries like cephalhaematoma, caput succedaneum, subgaleal haemorrhage are quite common in occurrence. Fractures of the skull are not very common birth injuries.

CEPHALHAEMATOMA

This haematoma develops on the surface of a cranial bone, often limited to parietal region and rarely over occipital bone. The swelling is visible several hours after birth as a soft one, not very tender. Very rarely cephalhaematoma is associated with skull fracture. The condition does not need any treatment as the swelling is absorbed gradually in two weeks to three months time depending upon the size of the

Birth Injuries

haematoma. Very rarely a massive haematoma causes big amount of blood loss necessitating in even blood transfusion. On very few occasions, there may be a sequel of bony protuberance over that area detected on X-ray as widening of the diploic space and calcification of haematoma. Sometimes, there is a marked hyperbilirubinemia where phototherapy may be necessary.

CAPUT SUCCEDANEUM

This diffuse oedematous and ecchymotic swelling of the scalp is present at birth. The swelling appears during vertex delivery, extend along the suture line and even crosses the midline. No specific treatment is required as the swelling disappears within a few days.

INTRA-CRANIAL HAEMORRHAGE

Intra-cranial haemorrhages in the newborn are associated with damage to the brain and may occur as subdural haemorrhage, subarachnoid haemorrhage, intra-cerebral haemorrhage and intra-ventricular haemorrhage.

Various precipitating factors and the signs detected in the affected baby help in establishing a clinical diagnosis. These are:

Subdural haemorrhage—This may be of acute or subacute or focal type occurring in a full-term baby, being delivered due to a precipitate or difficult labour. The subacute haemorrhage occurs 24 days after birth. Other varieties manifest few minutes to hours after birth. The features of acute subdural haemorrhage are stupor, rigidity to deviation of neck, bradycardia and opisthotonos. The condition may be fatal causing death. In focal cerebral syndrome, the baby presents with focal seizures, hemiparesis of focal nature and deviation of the eyes to the side of the lesion.

In subacute subdural haemorrhage occurring 24 days after birth, the onset is manifested with irritability, stupor, irregular respiration followed by brainstem compression.

Other varieties—subarachnoid, pre or interventricular and intracerebral haemorrhage occur in pre-term and low birth weight babies or in full-term babies following trauma.

The investigations to diagnose intracranial haemorrhages are:
1. Fundus examination—to detect haemorrhage in the fundus of the eye.
2. Lumbar puncture—to detect any change in the colour of the fluid, increased RBC and protein.
3. Subdural tap—in suspected subdural haemorrhage.
4. Cranial ultrasonography—to demonstrate periventricular or intraventricular haemorrhage, shift of midline structures and size of lateral ventricles.
5. Blood examination of total count, BT, CT, PCV, platelet count.
6. CT scan—Where the prognosis is bad due to increase in haemorrhage—to detect the site and extent of haemorrhage.

BIRTH FRACTURES

Fractures in the newborn babies may be observed at different sites. The fracture may occur with or without displacement or it may be an epiphyseal separation due to injury sustained during a difficult delivery. Fractures in pathological bones like those in osteogenesis imperfecta or in congenital pseudoarthrosis tibia have been described in separate chapters. The following fractures occur commonly in the newborn and need special mentioning.

Skull Fractures

Fractures in the skull may occur as (a) Linear fracture, (b) Depressed fracture and (c) Occipital osteodiastasis. However, the pliable nature of skull bone with wide open sutures protect the infant skull bone from fractures.

Linear Fracture

This linear crack in a skull is associated with extra and intra-cranial haemorrhage. The cause is a difficult delivery or foetopelvic disproportion. Usually no treatment is required except in complication like a leptomeningeal cyst formation.

Depressed Fracture

A palpable depression in the skull bone with or without occurrence of intra or extra-cranial haemorrhage is the usual mode of presentation. The cause is localised compression by forceps application or cephalopelvic disproportion. The diagnosed area of bone undergoes spontaneous elevation. Treatment by elevation of depression is necessary only when the depression is pronounced. If left untreated the latter presents as a depression or furrow in the adult life.

Occipital Osteodiastasis

The usual mode of presentation is separation of squamous part of occipital bone with or without damage to occipital sinus and cerebellum. The cause is forcible hyperextension of the neck during delivery of the trapped head in the pelvis in breech presentation. The condition is usually fatal.

Cervical Spine Injury

Excessive traction and torsional trauma during obstetric procedures may cause cervical spine injury at birth. This is due to weak cervical muscles and ligaments in the newborn unable to protect the cervical spine from trauma. Atlanto-occipital and atlanto-axial dislocations have been reported in the newborn. The hyperextension of the cervical spine seen in breech presentation may result in cervical cord injury during forcible breech extraction in vaginal delivery.[4]

Fracture of the Clavicle

Fracture of the clavicle due to birth trauma occurs in the midshaft of the bone and is caused usually by trauma by digital pressure on the bone while applying traction on the shoulders to deliver an after-coming head. The condition is usually diagnosed after about three weeks from the formation of a lump due to callus formation at the fracture site and from the X-ray taken on suspicion. No treatment is necessary except avoidance of pulling on the arm of the baby for the first-three or four weeks till the fracture consolidates.

Fracture of Shaft of the Humerus

Fracture of the shaft of the humerus occurs in the midshaft of the bone due to birth trauma while delivering an extended arm in breech presentation or during the delivery of impacted shoulders in a vertex presentation by applying axillary traction. The fracture site is angulated laterally due to the pull of the deltoid on the upper fragment.

The diagnosis is established by clinical examination. The motionless condition of the arm lying by the side of the baby raises suspicion of Erb's palsy, which is differentiated by the angulation of the humerus and the tenderness on its midshaft. Radiography confirms the diagnosis.

The treatment done by the author is simple splintage of the arm with a well-padded wooden or plastic spoon used by icecream vendors, which is folded on itself and made to proper size and then wrapped with the affected arm by further padding. The callus formation is usually within three weeks. The residual angulation is corrected automatically with time.

Fracture of Shaft of the Femur

Fracture shaft of the femur is not that uncommon birth injury and occurs usually at the upper-half of femur due to pull on the thigh with a rotational force during a breech delivery with extended leg. Even during extraction of a breech presentation by caesarean section, the fracture of the femoral shaft may occur. Here, the upper fragment is flexed anteriorly due to strong pull of the psoas muscle.

Treatment: As the callus formation is very early, the treatment is directed towards union of fracture without any complication like angulation and shortening. The method of strapping the affected thigh on the front of the baby's body with the hip flexed does correct the angulation, producing at times over correction with anterior angulation. Shortening often remains uncorrected. The best way to correct shortening and angulation is to apply traction along lower limbs by suspending the limbs from the crossbar of a birth fracture frame. The treatment is started from the day one and the frame is removed after 2 weeks, when there is enough callus formation.

EPIPHYSEAL SEPARATION

Epiphyseal separation in birth injuries due to difficult delivery like breech extraction takes place mostly in the lower femoral, upper and lower humeral epiphyses. The diagnosis is by swelling around the lower or upper end of the bone due to subperiosteal haematoma with tenderness on the swelling. The affected limb is almost immobile as the child avoids movements in that limb. Radiography will confirm the diagnosis. X-rays show displacement of fragments as is found in supracondylar fractures in children. The periosteum is lifted due to haematoma. The diagnosis of lower humeral epiphyseal separation is sometimes difficult till X-ray after two weeks, when subperiosteal bone formation is seen.

The treatment is by gentle manipulation to reduce the fragments as far as possible, as vigorous manipulation may cause vascular injury. In the lower limb, the plaster will be in semi-extended position and in the upper limb the plastering will be in a position of flexion keeping the forearm just above right-angle. The union of fracture is almost within three weeks. Slight displacement, which remains, is corrected automatically with age.

The separation of upper humeral epiphysis is diagnosed by local tenderness and immobility of the arm and is confirmed by X-ray. The treatment is by a simple sling or support on a small pillow.

BIRTH INJURIES OF THE BRACHIAL PLEXUS

Lesions of the brachial plexus are caused by violent forces applied during delivery of the baby. The lesions cause paralysis of part or whole of the upper limb. There may be some associated injuries of the ipsilateral clavicle, fracture separation of the proximal humeral growth plate, hip dysplasia, spasticity of the lower limbs or opposite upper limb due to haematomyelia or anoxia of the central nervous system.

Classification

There are three main types of paralysis of the upper limb according to the involvement of the components of the brachial plexus.
1. Upper arm type of Erb Duchenne—Caused by injury to the upper trunk at the junction of the fifth and sixth roots, known as Erb's point.
2. Lower arm type of Klumpke—Caused by injury to the eighth cervical and first thoracic nerve roots.
3. Paralysis of the entire arm—Caused by injury to all the components of the brachial plexus.

Incidence and Risk Factors

Brachial plexus injuries occur in 0.4 to 2.5 per 1000 live births.

The risk factors at birth are (i) breech presentation, (ii) prolonged labour, (iii) shoulder dystocia, when one shoulder is trapped behind the symphysis pubis, (iv) cephalopelvic disproportion, (v) excessive birth weight of the baby.

Etiology

The brachial plexus injury is caused by forced stretching of one or more components or whole of the plexus. The stretching is common during delivery of the head in breech presentation by strong traction of the trunk causing excessive lateral flexion of the neck of the baby. In vertex presentation, stretching is caused by strong traction necessary to free a shoulder trapped behind the symphysis pubis. Similarly, stretching of the head and neck during delivery of a baby with breech presentation even by caesarean section may cause brachial plexus injury.

Pathology

The brachial plexus injury will cause paresis or paralysis of the upper limb according to the nature of nerve injury from mild, moderate to severe, i.e. neuropraxia to axonotmesis. In milder form of injury, there is some perineural oedema and haemorrhage with early recovery in 3 months time. In moderate variety the stretching is more causing both intraneural and extraneural bleeding with tear of some of the nerve fibres. The recovery is usually complete in 2 years. In the severe type, there will be complete tear or avulsion of the brachial plexus with practically no chance of recovery except when early repair is undertaken within 2 to 3 months after birth. The disruption of the nerve roots when occur may take place at the intervertebral foramen or there may be avulsion from the spinal cord.

Clinical Presentation and Diagnosis

There can be some tale-tell evidence on the neonate helping diagnosis of brachial plexus injury. There can be supraclavicular swelling or ecchymosis with cephalhaematoma suggesting forceps injury. The findings of Horner's syndrome like ptosis, miosis, enophthalmos suggest first dorsal nerve root with sympathetic fibre injury. If the breathing is normal, there cannot be paralysis of the diaphragm, i.e. injury to the phrenic nerve. Fractures associated with brachial plexus injury are ipsilateral fracture of the clavicle, fracture of the humeral shaft or upper humeral epiphyseal separation and occasionally dislocation of the shoulder. The symptoms as above and X-ray showing one of the fractures described will suggest brachial plexus injury.

The condition is to be differentiated from osteomyelitis of the humerus or the clavicle or from septic arthritis of the shoulder when the ipsilateral upper limb will be devoid of normal motion—a pseudoparalysis. In brachial plexus injury, the Moro reflex will be absent, which will not be the case in pseudoparalysis. Besides, there will be pain, tenderness, oedema, and swelling of osteomyelitis or septic arthritis, which will be absent in plexus injury.

Besides plain X-ray of cervical spine, myelogram and MRI should be done to know the exact pathology and the level of injury.

Treatment

Surgical repair of disrupted upper plexus roots with sutures in four babies with brachial plexus injuries was done between 2 and 6 months of birth by Kennedy[5,6] in 1903. The procedure was considered as unrewarding for quite sometime. After a lapse of seven decades, there is a revival of early surgical repair of brachial plexus injury between two and three months of birth of babies by Solonen et al[7] in three cases. They have taken the help of electroneuromyography and microsurgical nerve reconstruction. Surgery was undertaken when repeated clinical and electroneuromyographic examinations showed no improvement and total disruption of at least one nerve root was found. The procedure was repair with free sural grafts. In a follow-up of 15 to 33 months they found improvement in deltoid, biceps and external rotators of the upper arm to a certain extent. Although Solonen et al used sural nerve grafts for repair, they have recommended direct neurorrhaphy also. Gilbert et al[8] used intercostal nerve grafts for repair at 3 months of age when there was no return of elbow flexion and shoulder abduction. He did not recommend microsurgical repair in partial paralysis.

However, in most of the cases conservative treatment was followed keeping the arm in a position of abduction and external rotation when the nerves of brachial plexus were not in tension. This practice is now condemned in favour of passive exercises to retain range of motion of the shoulder, elbow, forearm and wrist and to prevent contractures. Electrical stimulation of nerves is used but rigid splinting is not used. However, when the upper limb is absolutely flail due to nerve injury, the hand and wrist are splinted in functional position in between physiotherapy.

The treatment of residual fixed medial rotation-adduction deformity is done by lateral rotation osteotomy of the humerus. For medial rotation contracture of the shoulder subscapularis recession at its origin is recommended.[9] The latter when associated with weakness of lateral rotators of the shoulder is treated with transfer of latissimus dorsi to the rotator cuff as an additional procedure. A flail shoulder will need arthrodesis at around the time of skeletal maturity, provided scapulothoracic and scapular elevators and the trapezius muscles are of sufficient motor power.

Prognosis

In neonates with brachial plexus injury recovery will be somewhat satisfactory if the damage is minimum, but in those with moderate or severe damage, recovery will be satisfactory in only 8 per cent cases.[10] Maximum recovery takes place spontaneously within one and a half and two years of age of the baby. The residual paralysis may cause adduction internal rotation contracture of the shoulder or in extreme variety a flail limb.[11]

REFERENCES

1. Kulkarni ML. Manual of Neonatology. New Delhi: Jaypee Brothers Medical Publishers (P) Ltd.p.321.
2. Agarwal S, et al. Indian Pediatrics 1978;15:1005.
3. Shulmann ST, Madden JD, Esterly JR. Transection of Spinal Cord - A rare obstetrical complication of cephalic delivery. Arch Dis Child 1971;46:291-94.
4. Breman MJ, Abrams TF. Neural spinal cord transection secondary to intrauterine hypertension of the neck in breech presentation J Pediatr 1974;84:734-37.
5. Kennedy R. Suture of the Brachial plexus in birth paralysis of the upper extremity. Br Med J 1903;I: 298-301, 1903, quoted by Solonen et al in J Ped Orthop. 1981;1:367-70.
6. Kennedy R. Further notes on the treatment of birth paralysis of the upper extremity by suture of the fifth and sixth cervical nerves. Br Med J 1904;II: 1065-68, quoted by Solomen et al in J Ped Orthop 1981;1: 367-70.
7. Solomen KA, Telaranta T, Ryoppy S. Early reconstruction of birth injuries of the brachial plexus. J Ped Orthop 1981;1:367-70.
8. Gilbert A, Razaboni R, Amar-Khodja S. Indications and results of brachial plexussurgery in obstetrical palsy. Orthop Clin North Am 1988;19:91.
9. Carlioz H, Brahimi L. La place dela desinsertion interne du son-scapulaire dans le traitement de la paralysic obstetrical du membre superieur chez l'enfant. Ann Chir Infant 1971;12: 159, quoted by Tachdjian MO, Clinical Pediatric Orthopedics: The art of diagnosis and principles of management, Stanford, Appleton and Lange, 296.
10. Wickstrom J. Birth injuries of the brachial plexus. Treatment of defects in the shoulder. Clin Orthop 1969;23: 187-96.
11. Wickstrom J, Haslam ET, Hutchinson RH. The surgical management of residual deformities of the shoulder following birth injuries of the brachial plexus. J Bone Joint Surg (Am) 1955;37:27-36.

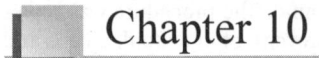

Chapter 10

Congenital Developmental Anomalies of the Extremities in the Neonate

Keywords: Genetics, environmental and iatrogenic factors, sometimes hereditary factors as cause – two types – terminal and intercalary – congenital constriction band syndrome.

Proper development of the skeleton requires a total harmony between the power or the genetic contribution and the passage the embryonic condition. Any disharmony will lead to suffering of the passenger—the offspring, in the form of a deficiency evident at birth. The exact cause of limb anomalies is not known. Most of the abnormalities occur sporadically; hereditary factor is observed in a few cases. No familial occurrences and no known injuries have been found. However, the following factors have been put forward as the cause.

ETIOLOGY

Genetic Factor

Genes in ovum or sperm are responsible for the transmission of specific anomalies according to Mendel's law, which indicates involvement with skeletal deficiency of a large number of offspring in case of dominant inheritance, whereas recessive factor produces infrequent occurrence of anomalies.

Embryonic Environment

The defect develops within seven weeks of intrauterine life—the period within which the embryo develops into a recognizable human form. After the limb buds appear on the lateral body wall from the tissues of the condensed mesoderm of lateral plate in the 4th post-ovulatory week, the limbs develop in a proximodistal sequence. From the condensation of lateral plate mesoderm the skeletal elements develop in a sequence of first chondrification and then ossification, and the muscles develop *in situ*. Endochondral bone formation takes place within five to seven weeks of intrauterine life. The motor fibres grow from the spinal cord into this unsegmented lateral plate and are arranged in a segmental pattern. Experimental production of skeletal defects was shown by Duraiswami through his classic experiments by injecting insulin in chick embryo.[1]

Iatrogenic Factor

Maternal thalidomide ingestion causes defects of limbs. Hamanishi[2] found association of absence of tibia with defects in other limbs due to thalidomide intake, compared to association of absence of fibula with naturally occurring defects.

Anomalies of Development

The anomalies to be described below develop within seven weeks of embryonic life. Increase in skeletal elements like polydactyly or failure of development leading to limb deficiency, like hemimelia to complete amelia or phocomelia all take place within this period.

Two types of congenital limb deficiencies have been described—terminal and intercalary. The deficiency may be termed amelia which means absence of one or more limbs and hemimelia is the lack of distal part of a limb, e.g. a forearm or a hand or a leg or a foot, with a normally developed proximal part and thirdly congenital amputation stump. The hemimelia may be complete or incomplete. The deficiency may involve all four extremities or more frequently one or two may be involved. The phocomelia (Greek phoko means seal)—an intercalary deficiency is marked by incomplete development of the middle part of a limb, e.g. the hand or foot is attached directly to the arm or the thigh (Figs 10.1 and 10.2). If the

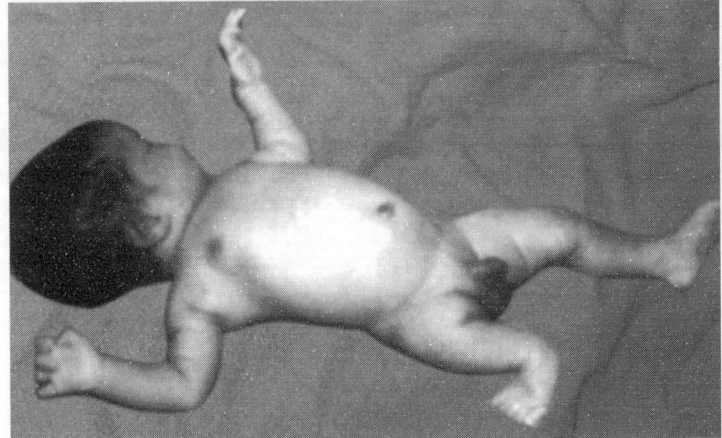

Fig. 10.1: Intercalary congenital limb deficiency showing incomplete development of middle part of right lower limb—the foot being attached at a higher level compared to the normal left side

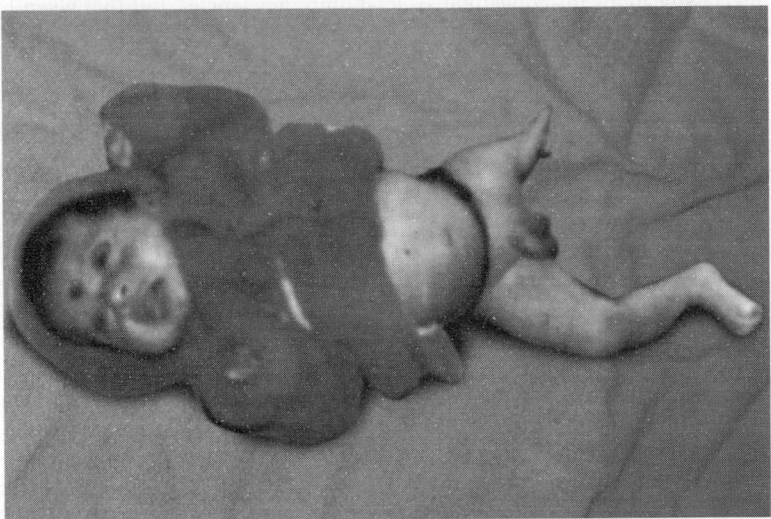

Fig. 10.2: Phocomelia in the left lower limb

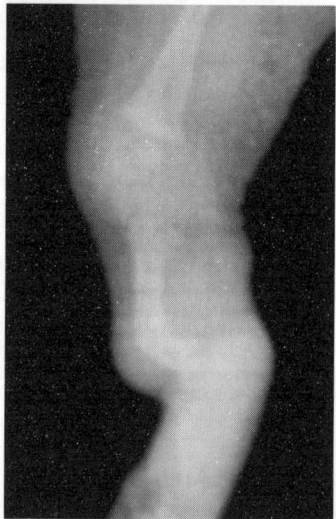

Fig. 10.3: Radiograph of complete paraxial hemimelia of fibula with short leg, bowed tibia and deformed foot

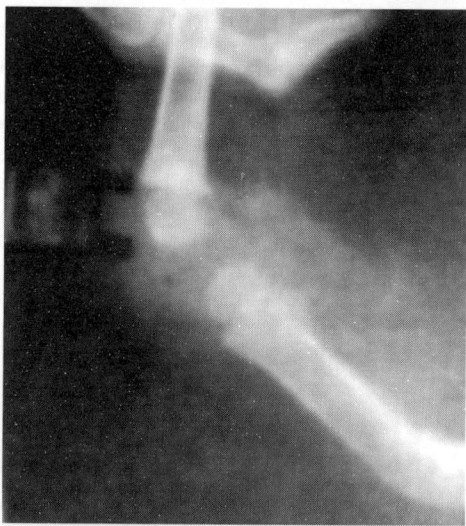

Fig. 10.4: Radiograph of the same patient as in Figure 10.3 at a later age with some straightening of the short tibia

anomaly involves pre- or post-axial part of the limb and the area distal to involvement fail to develop, remainder of the limb develops as paraxial deformity (Figs 10.3 and 10.4). The chance of involvement of subsequent children or in the children of the affected individual is very remote.

CLASSIFICATION OF LIMB DEFICIENCIES

There are many classifications for congenital skeletal limb deficiencies, but that given by Frantz and O'Rahilly[3] is universally accepted:

Terminal deficiencies		Intercalary deficiencies	
There are no unaffected parts distal to and in line with the deficient portion		Middle portion of limb is deficient but proximal and distal portions are present	
Transverse Defect extends transversely across the width of the limb	Paraxial-Only the pre-axial or post-axial portion of limb is absent	Transverse-Entire central portion of limb absent with foreshortening	Paraxial–Segmental absence of pre-axial or post-axial limb segments—intact proximal and distal

A definite entity—amniotic bands, have been found as the known cause of pre-natal amputation and the symptom complex is known as Streeter syndrome. The constricting bands may produce obstruction of venous drainage with resulting oedema or in more severe cases as deep clefts in soft tissues. In the very severe and rare form occurring late in intrauterine life amputation of extremity may occur and the amputated extremity is delivered with the body.

Kino[4] after reproduction of the syndrome in rat foetuses by amniocentesis opined that the malformations were due to excessive contraction of the uterine muscles during pregnancy causing haemorrhage from blood vessels of the digital rays. He observed the time of damage at about six weeks of intrauterine development of the foetus.

Management

Nothing is more challenging than managing a limb deficient infant into a fit child capable of day to day normal work. The biggest challenge the surgeon faces is to make the parents aware of the true situation and the ultimate outcome. The pros and cons of two different methods of treatment are to be discussed with the parents before coming to a decision. The first one—an early amputation although quicker in achieving results, has to be done at appropriate time for the proper management of the baby. The second one—the reconstructive surgery is time consuming, takes a very long time to finish and at times may turn up into a hurried final work out because of the telling effect on recipients for long procedures performed for a totally uncertain result.

Amputation

The time of amputating the upper limb specially from forearm or wrist is around six months when the child learns sitting and brings both the hands closer to each other and use them together. This helps in a better prosthesis fitting. For the lower limb, the average time for an amputation is around ten months just before the child learns walking. Not only the technical aspect of prosthesis fitting is better but also the psychic trauma is less with this work out.

Regarding prosthetic fitting in children one has to consider the age of the child. As young children suffer from immature balance or the knee is not needed in a toddler's first above-knee prosthesis, articulated knees are used skillfully at around the age of three years.

Reconstructive Surgery

This is often multiple in nature. After a child learns walking reconstructive correction of certain deformities is better maintained. The fusion procedures are best done when the bone anlage is well ossified.

The difficulty arises in selecting between the above two procedures in some of the situations. The best example is fibular hemimelia when a Syme amputation at around ten months of age takes the child to almost normal activities, even in sports, except that he or she will have to adjust mentally with a prothesis devoid of a normal foot. When a patient does not want amputation, the reconstructive procedure is usually undertaken late, in adolescence, putting the child into a lengthy but modern limb-lengthening procedure.

CONGENITAL CONSTRICTION BAND SYNDROME (STREETER SYNDROME)

This congenital constriction, of the soft tissue of the leg and toes usually and of the upper limb rarely, is present at birth and may completely encircle the leg (Fig. 10.5), toes or fingers and forearm. Amniotic bands have been said as the cause of this constriction as Streeter syndrome, as mentioned before. The constriction may extend from the skin through the subcutaneous tissue upto the deep fascia causing oedema of the tissues distal to the constriction but having no effect on the underlying bone (Fig. 10.6). There are reports of fractures of bones at the site of constriction, which are very rare in incidence. The fractures heal after successful treatment of constriction.

The treatment of constriction is removal of it by surgery in early infancy. The operation is Z-plasty operation—one or multiple at stages, depending upon the extent of—encirclement of the constriction, i.e. partial or complete encirclement. The lengthening of the constriction throughout its circumference gives a better look to the area with gradual improvement of oedema distal to the constriction.

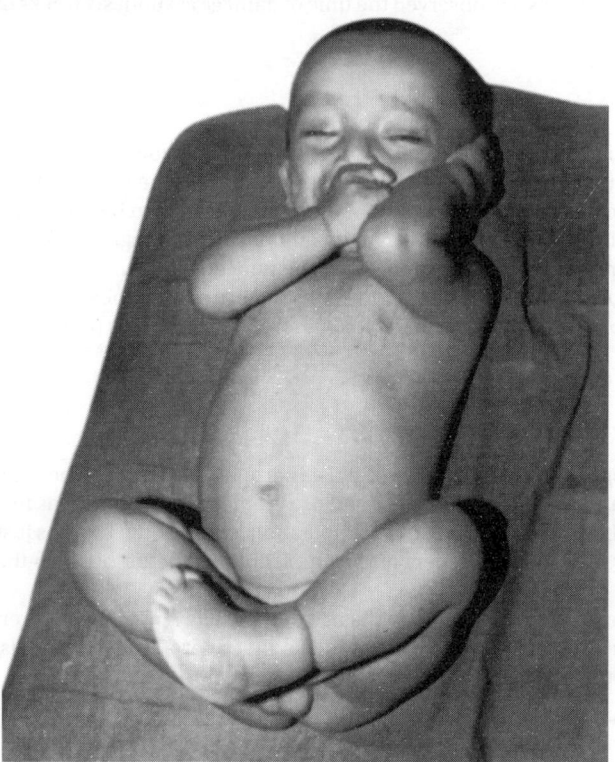

Fig. 10.5: Congenital constriction ring completely encircling the left leg

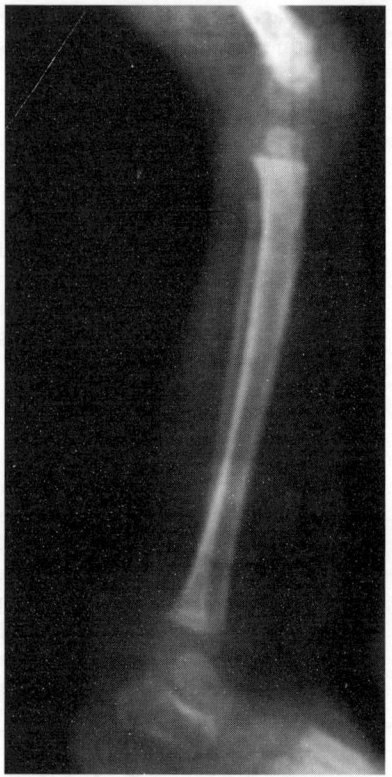

Fig. 10.6: Radiograph showing congenital constriciton band having no effect on the underlying bone

REFERENCES

1. Duraiswai PK. Experimental causation of congenital skeletal defects in orthopaedic surgery. J Bone Joint Surg 1952;34B:646.
2. Hemanishi C. Congenital short femur. Clinical, genetic and epidemiological comparison of the naturally occurring condition with that caused by thalidomide. J Bone Joint Surg (Br) 1980;62B:307-20.
3. Frantz CH, O'Rahilly R. J Bone Joint Surg 1961;43A:1202.
4. Kino Y. Clinical and experimental studies of the congenital constriction band syndrome, with an emphasis on its etiology. J Bone Joint Surg. 1975;57A:636.

Chapter 11

Neonatal Rickets

Keywords: Rickets in neonates is manifested by multiple fractures, osteoporosis, bending of bones, high alkaline phosphates, low serum calcium and slightly low phosphorus level. Low dietary calcium in a preterm baby is often the cause.

Rickets in a neonate, specially in a low birth weight baby, born after a very short gestational period (28-34 weeks) of the mother, is of a severe degree, as these babies are very prone to develop the condition.

ETIOLOGY

The cause of neonatal rickets may be one or multiple. Insufficient dietary calcium specially in a preterm baby is often the cause, because, as the gestational age progresses the absorption of calcium also increases. Sometimes due to improper absorption of vitamin D, the serum concentration of 25 hydroxy vitamin D is not maintained. The cause of this poor absorption is decreased absorption of fat and presence of lesser quantity of the bile acids.[1] Sometimes the hydroxylation of vitamin D in the liver is poor or the conversion of hydroxy vitamin D to dihydroxy vitamin D in the kidney is limited due to immaturity of the alpha-hydroxylase enzyme system responsible for the conversion. Even after proper conversion to dihydroxy vitamin D, the responsive organs like the intestine, the kidney and the bone function well only when the dihydroxy vitamin D is present in a high dose.

Infant's vitamin D level in the circulation depends upon the maternal circulatory vitamin D. The placenta has got a role in the transport of maternal vitamin D to the foetus. Recent studies show the existence of a calcium pump mechanism in the villus brush border of the human placenta.

There is a sudden stoppage of the maternal calcium to the newborn baby as the placental connection goes off. The newborn baby, therefore, depends upon dietary calcium, good intestinal transport and metabolism within the body. The infant gets the advantage of synthesis of vitamin D through skin after birth.

Often neonatal rickets is found among underprivileged classes because of dietary deficiency of vitamin D and calcium in the mothers, specially when they have repeated pregnancies.

CLINICAL, BIOCHEMICAL AND RADIOGRAPHIC FEATURES

The rickets in these babies is manifested clinically by the presence of multiple fractures and bone deformities in some of them with biochemical changes and radiographic features corroborating them. The alkaline phosphatase which is 400 IU in a normal baby is raised[2] to 576 to 1955 with a mean value of 1010. The serum phosphorus value is slightly low, the normal value being 4 to 6 mgm per cent. The serum calcium level is also

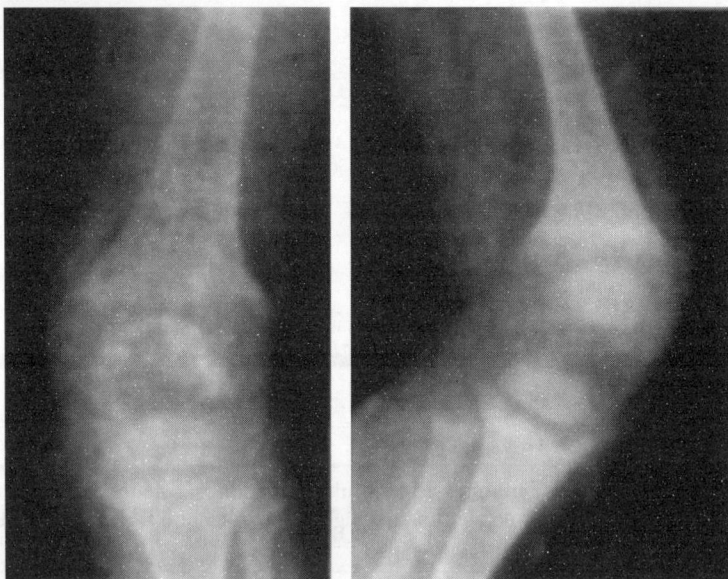

Fig. 11.1: Irregularity of the metaphyseal end of diaphysis and a widened clear zone between the epiphyses and the diaphysis in osteoporotic bones shown in a case of neonatal rickets

low 6.8 to 8.1 mgm per cent, the normal being 8.6 to 10.5 mgm per cent. The parathormone level in pre-term rachitic babies is raised to 25 to 65, the mean being 40 microequivalents per ml. The normal parathormone level in babies is 2 to 10 microequivalents per ml. The serum 25 hydroxy vitamin D is around 10 mg/ml in the normal babies, but in pre-term rachitic babies, the level is as low as 3.6 mg/ml, the range being 2 to 6 mg/ml.

Radiographically these babies show generalised osteoporosis, irregularity of the metaphyseal end of diaphysis with a widened clear zone between the epiphysis and the diaphysis, bending of bones and fractures (Fig. 11.1).

MANAGEMENT

Prevention of rickets among low-birth weight infants is very important in developing countries. In the antenatal care mothers should be treated with vitamin D and calcium to improve dietary deficiency.

Low birth weight babies of short-term gestation should get 800 to 1000 IU of vitamin D per day to prevent rickets.

Low birth weight babies when treated with large doses of vitamin D_2 (4000 IU per day) show an increase in utilisation and high levels of hydroxy vitamin D_3, which are useful for bone mineralisation. The production of dihydroxy vitamin D_3 in the kidney is increased with large doses of vitamin D and the presence of high serum hydroxy vitamin D_3 level. The presence of growth hormone, prolactin, thyroid hormones and corticosteroids help in the process. Increased parathormone level in the absence of phosphate and calcium help in the production of dihydroxy vitamin D_3.

REFERENCES

1. Koo WWK, Sherman R, Swaroop P. Fractures and rickets in very low birth weight infants – conservative management and outcome. J Pediatr Orthop 1989;9:326.
2. Udani PM. Textbook of pediatrics. New Delhi: Jaypee Brothers Medical Publishers (P) Ltd. 1998;1:639.

Section 2: Lower Limb Anomalies

Chapter 12

Bent Bones in a Neonate

Keywords: Bent bones in a neonate may be kyphoscoliosis of both tibia and fibula or anterolateral bowing of the tibia or the fibula – rarely in others the tibia is short and bent with absence of fibula and outer two toes

Bending of bones when found in the neonatal period may happen as a part of generalised deformity (neonatal rickets) or may be localised to a bone.

Localised bent bones of the leg will be discussed now and the generalised form has been described in the previous chapter.

The bent bones of the leg may show bowing post-eromedially involving both tibia and fibula forming a complex deformity of Kyphoscoliosis or it may predominantly involve tibia and sometimes fibula forming an antero-lateral bowing. The latter may ultimately turn into a fracture at the bent area producing pseudoarthrosis of tibia. Sometimes in another condition, the tibia is short and bent with absence of fibula and outer two toes.

CONGENITAL KYPHOSCOLIOSIS TIBIA AND FIBULA

The deformity is present at birth with postero-medial bowing of the tibia and the fibula having the foot placed in calcaneo valgus position. The bowing is prominent at the junction of the middle and distal thirds often with a dimple in the skin at the apex of the deformity. The calf muscles are sometimes found atrophied. The calcaneo valgus deformity of the foot is associated with contracture of the tibialis anterior, extensor digitorum longus, peroneus brevis and tertius muscles. The tibia and fibula are shorter than the contralateral tibia and fibula by an average of 1.2 cm in infancy to 4.1 cm in adulthood. The deformity is almost always unilateral.

Etiology

Although the cause of the deformity is not known a developmental defect taking place in the embryonic period has been incriminated. No hereditary or environmental cause *in utero* has been found.

Imaging Findings

Both AP and lateral X-rays show identical nature of deformity in the tibia and the fibula, the medial bowing is prominent in the AP and posterior bowing is well-evident in the lateral view. The cortices on the

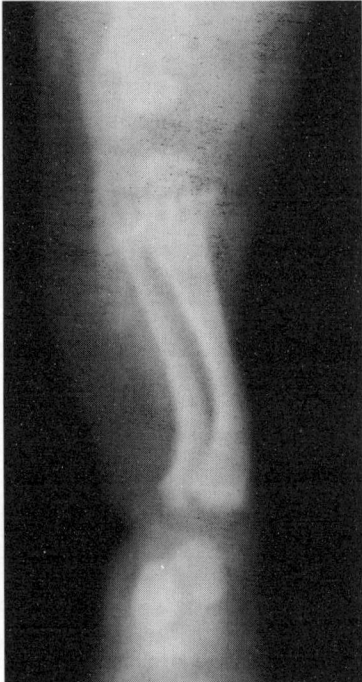

Fig. 12.1: Congenital kyphoscoliosis of tibia fibula with delayed ossification of distal tibial and fibular epiphyses—the ankle, subtalar and midtarsal joints are normal

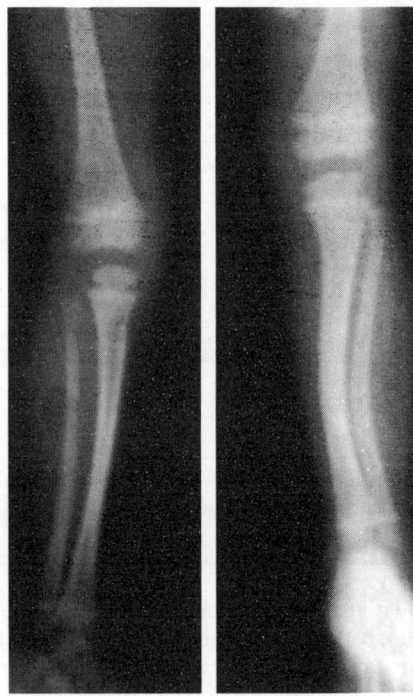

Fig. 12.2: Spontaneous correction of kyphoscoliosis of tibia fibular bone growth

anterior and the lateral surfaces of the tibia and the fibula are thickened. The intramedullary canal is not narrowed and there is no intramedullary sclerosis. Ossification of the distal tibial and fibular epiphyses is delayed. The ankle, subtalar and the midtarsal joints are normal (Fig. 12.1).

Natural History

There is a spontaneous correction of bowing with bone growth (Fig. 12.2). There is about fifty per cent correction of deformity by 2 years of age. The rate of correction is slowed down after the 3rd year. Posterior angulation is corrected more readily than the medial bowing and the tibial correction is quicker than the fibular improvement. The calcaneovalgus deformity is also corrected fully leaving a residual defect of planovalgus of the foot during adolescence. The limb length disparity at skeletal maturity is at an average of 4.1 cm.

Treatment

As the correction of deformity of leg is spontaneous attention is paid to the treatment of the calcanovalgus deformity. In mild deformity stretching in opposite direction corrects the defect, which should be started in the neonatal period. In moderate to severe varieties correction by serial casts is necessary followed after correction by stretching at day time and splintage at night.

Orthosis for bowing of leg is superfluous as the correction is spontaneous. If the posterior angulation is more than 30° after the age of four years, correction by anterior and lateral angulation osteotomy is necessary.

Limb length disparity is corrected by either stapling of contralateral upper tibial and fibular epiphyses if the shortening at 6 to 8 years of age is less than 4 cm; and by leg lengthening at around 8 to 10 years of age, if the disparity is more than 5 cm.

For residual flat foot, exercises and foot orthosis are good enough. Occasional severe cases need surgical correction.

Limb length disparity is corrected by either stapling of contralateral upper tibial and fibular epiphyses if the shortening at 6 to 8 years of age is less than 4 cm; and by leg lengthening at around 8 to 10 years of age, if the disparity is more than 5 cm.

For residual flat foot, exercises and foot orthosis are good enough. Occasional severe cases need surgical correction.

REFERENCES

1. Koo WWK, Sherman R, Swaroop P. Fractures and rickets in very low birth weight infants - conservative management and outcome. J Pediatr Orthop 1989;9:326.
2. Udani PM. Textbooks of Pediatrics. New Delhi: Jaypee Brothers Medical Publishers (P) Ltd. 1998;1:639.

Chapter 13

Congenital Pseudoarthrosis of the Tibia and Fibula

Keywords: Congenital pseudoarthrosis of tibia - a rare condition of anterolateral bowing of tibia with sometimes pathological fracture-very difficult to heal with treatment-classified by Boyd into six different types.

CONGENITAL PSEUDOARTHROSIS OF TIBIA

Congenital pseudoarthrosis of tibia is a rare condition of antero-lateral bowing of tibia with or without a defect at the apex of the bowing, having an incidence of 1 in 1,00000 live births.[1] The condition appears at birth with different modes of presentation. Boyd has classified six different types.[2]

Type I presents with anterior bowing of the junction of middle and lower third of tibia and narrowing of medullary canal at that region at birth with some atrophy and shortening of the leg. This is the incipient type (Fig. 13.1).

Type II occurs at birth with anterior bowing and an hourglass constriction of the tibia. A fracture appears at the site of narrowing either spontaneously or after a minor trauma very rarely at birth but usually before the age of 1½ to 2 years when the child crawls or stand. This is the most frequent type and is often associated with neurofibromatosis. In this dysplastic type, the X-ray shows hourglass narrowing with or without fracture, the medullary canal being partially or completely obliterated by sclerosis. The bone ends at the fracture site are covered by hamartomatous fibrous tissue. Hence, the incidence of

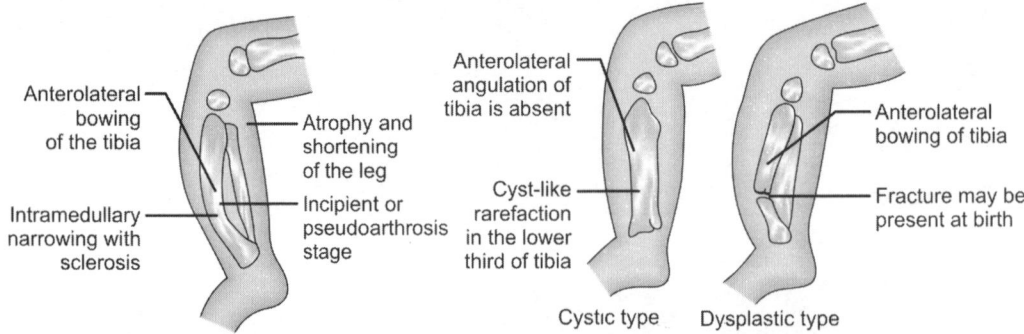

Fig. 13.1: Congenital pseudoarthrosis of the tibia in neonate depicted in a diagram presenting incipient, cystic and dysplastic types of which the dysplastic type shows a fracture

non-union of fracture following treatment is very high specially during the growth period. Fibula is often involved as well.

Type III presents at birth with cystic appearances at the junction of middle and distal thirds of tibia—the cystic type. The anterolateral angulation gradually develops in the first six months of life. The pathologic fracture develops at around 8 months of age of the baby. The cysts are well visible in the X-ray usually at the site of narrowing of the tibia but sometimes in the fibula also when there is some narrowing of that bone. As this type is not associated with neurofibromatosis the chances of non-union of fracture following treatment is infrequent.

Type IV: Here, the bone shows a sclerotic segment with slight anterolateral bowing at the junction of middle and distal thirds of tibia with partial or complete obliteration of the medullary cavity in the X-ray. There is no fracture at birth but there is development of a break in the anterior cortex in early childhood with gradual extension of the break through the sclerotic bone. Gradually there develops a pseudoarthrosis. Usually the fracture heals well if treated early, before the fracture becomes complete.

Type V: This may be called a variant of type II with dysplastic involvement of both the tibia and the fibula. The prognosis is good if the fibula is only involved.

Type VI: Here, the pseudoarthrosis is due to an intraosseous neurofibroma or Schwannoma. The condition is extremely rare.

Treatment

In the neonatal period the object of treatment is to prevent stress fracture in the type II variety by applying a POP back slab. When the pseudoarthrosis is established at a later date surgery in the form of double-onlay bone grafting or Ilizarov technique of compression by bone transport lengthening the proximal metaphysis or application of a bypass posterior graft or reconstruction by free vascularised fibular transplant from opposite side is undertaken according to the situation. As the union is weak an inserted IM nail gives stability to the affected bone. But, inspite of repeated surgery a pseudoarthrosis of tibia may not unite and the ultimate treatment may even be amputation.

CONGENITAL PSEUDOARTHROSIS OF FIBULA

This condition is not evident in the neonatal period. When the pseudoarthrosis is developed at a later date, the area of fibula, which is usually distal metaphyseal-diaphyseal region, shows a swelling with lateral bowing along with eversion deformity of hindfoot and slight shortening of the leg. There is concomitant involvement of the tibia and gradual development of ankle valgus with riding up of the lateral malleolus.

The treatment is excision of pseudoarthrosis, intramedullary fixation and bone grafting. Ankle valgus also needs treatment by adoption of surgical procedure of distal tibiofibular synostosis or in established case by supramelleolar osteotomy.

REFERENCES

1. Clinical Pediatric Orthopedics - the art of diagnosis and principles of management by Mihran O Tachdjian, 1997, 133.
2. Campbell's operative orthopedics; ed. By A.H. Crenschaw; (7th ed) CV Mosby Co., 1987;4:2670.

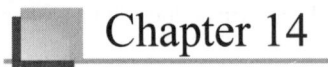

Congenital Lower Limb Defects

Keywords: Congenital lower limb defects are congenital short femur, congenital longitudinal deficiency of the tibia and the fibula – basic treatment is centralisation of the existing bone – correction of proximal and distal joint deformities – correction of shortening of limb length.

Lower limb defects of congenital origin may be of different types, as discussed in a chapter before. Here, I would like to discuss some of the specific problems like congenital defects of the femur and congenital longitudinal deficiency of the tibia, congenital longitudinal deficiency of the fibula and congenital tibio-fibular diastasis. Congenital femoral focal deficiency and congenital foot defects are discussed in separate chapters. Congenital deficiency of lower limbs are found to have instability of the knee.[1] Johansson and Aparisi[2] have detected absence of one or both cruciate ligaments in such conditions.

CONGENITAL DEFECTS OF THE FEMUR

The anomalies of the femur of congenital origin may be congenital short femur or femoral hypoplasia, which will be discussed here. The congenital abnormality with marked osseous defect is designated as congenital femoral focal deficiency and will be described separately. The same dysplastic or genetic cause may produce either of these defects as is evidenced by the presence of congenital femoral focal deficiency in one limb and hypoplasia in the other femur. The differences between the two seem to be a matter of inhibition of growth and the defects of ossification in some parts of the proximal femur.

Severe types of congenital femoral defects are associated with other skeletal limb defects like absence of tibia or fibula. Often femoral and tibial defects are associated with deficiency of the radius and fibular anomalies having association with ulnar deficiency.

Gillespie and Torode's[3] classification which conforms to the plan of treatment is followed here. Their classification of Group I includes congenital short femur, where knee and hip are relatively normal, can have a good prognosis following limb equalisation.

Group II with proximal femoral focal deficiency will have a defective hip and an almost useless knee.

Congenital Short Femur (Femoral Hypoplasia)

Congenital short femur is a condition with smaller length of the femur compared to the normal side, developed from femoral hypoplasia. Broadly speaking, there are two varieties, one without coxa vara and the other associated with coxa vara, developing from the region of trochanter or sub-trochanteric region.

The first variety presents with a short thigh mostly of unilateral occurrence, sometimes associated with lateral bowing in a neonate with its lower limb laterally rotated having limitation of medial rotation. The cruciate ligaments are often absent. Delayed ossification of the capital femoral epiphysis in a short femur is the characteristic radiological finding. But the ultimate development of hip is normal. The area of lateral bowing, when present, is in the midshaft of the femur having an area of cortical thickening and sometimes narrowing of medullary canal.[4] According to severity of radiological changes the deformity is identified by Hamanishi[5] into four grades starting from the first grade of simple hypoplasia of femur to the second variety with slight lateral bowing of femur; the third having lateral bowing due to a transverse sub-trochanteric ossification defect and fourth grade with a decreased neck-shaft angle. The bowing corrects with age leaving an occasional tell-tale evidence of sclerosis of the shaft.

The ultimate limb length inequality at maturity is predictable in this condition as the ratio of the longitudinal growth of the short femur to that of the femur of the healthy side remains the same throughout growth. The limb is 10 per cent shorter than the normal limb at the maturity unless there is associated shortening in tibia.

The correction is by surgery if the inequality is more than 2 cm. Surgery is by epiphysiodesis of the opposite distal femur if the shortening is between 2 to 5 cm, and in shortening above 5 cm. the correction is by leg lengthening. Sometimes, there is a delay in ossification at the site of distraction of callus due to abnormality in the quality of the bone of the shaft as revealed in the preoperative X-ray. Some degree of protection by orthosis for quite sometime in the post-lengthening period is necessary in those cases. Less than 2 cm. shortening is corrected by raised shoes.

Congenital Short Femur with Coxa Vara

This variety of short femur with coxa vara is often mistaken in the neonatal period with DDH due to the limitation of abduction present in both the conditions. The presence of limitation of medial rotation in this condition identifies this from DDH. The short femur with coxa vera is due to delayed ossification of cartilaginous upper one-third of the femur which is ossified at about 2 years of age. The result is a gap in the X-ray between the upper femur, which looks bulbous,[6] and the acetabulum, which is usually normal in appearance. The varus is from the trochanteric or subtrochanteric region, the femur below showing sclerosis of the shaft with narrowing of the medullary canal. Occasionally, the acetabulum is dysplastic. An ultrasonography or MRI displays the changes in the upper femur.

The treatment will depend upon the progress of varus and shortening. If the varus goes on increasing a valgus osteotomy is recommended. The shortening of femur is more in this condition and the predictable shortening of limb is 30 per cent of the normal. Therefore, femoral lengthening here is done in two stages within pubertal age.

CONGENITAL LONGITUDINAL DEFICIENCY OF THE TIBIA

The condition is evident at birth and presents in three different forms. They are classified according to severity into those different types by Kalamchi and Dawe.[7] The first type, the type I is the worst and rare with absence of whole of tibia (tibial agenesis). This will be described separately. In type II only the distal half of the tibia is absent, the foot assuming the position of adduction and inversion like a clubfoot with slightly diminished leg length. The knee joint shows a flexion deformity of about 25 to 30° and a high riding proximal fibula. The type III shows a hypoplastic tibia with diastasis of the distal tibiofibular syndesmosis. The leg is short with a relatively normal knee. This was first described by Tuli and Verma[8] in 1972 and is a distinct entity.[9]

According to Jones et al[10] there are four different clinical and radiological types. In the type 1a the tibia is not seen and the lower femoral epiphysis is hypoplastic. The type 1b shows normal lower femoral epiphysis with absent tibia (Fig. 14.1). In the type 2, the distal tibia is absent whereas in type 3 the proximal tibia is not seen. In type 4, the tibia is short and there is distal tibiofibular diastasis (Fig. 14.2). The fibula is always intact. The foot is mostly normal or may show diplopodia in some or rarely polydactyly.

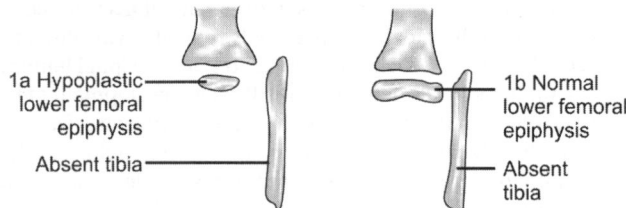

Fig. 14.1: Congenital longitudinal deficiency of the tibia—absent tibia in types 1a and 1b

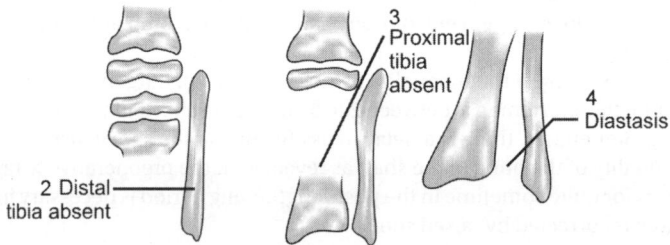

Fig. 14.2: Congenital longitudinal deficiency of the tibia—distal tibia absent in type 2, proximal tibia absent in type 3 and tibio-fibular diastasis in type 4

Tibial Agenesis

The condition was first described by Otto[11] in 1841. This is a complete intercalary longitudinal paraxial hemimelia.[12] It is considered as the rarest of congenital deformities occurring 1 in lac live-births and according to Kalamchi and Dawe's classification is type I.[13] As to the cause of tibial agenesis a family tendency has been incriminated.

Clinical Features

Tibial agenesis can be either unilateral or bilateral. At birth equinovarus deformity of the foot with knee flexion deformity having the fibular head at much higher level and congenital anomalies of other limbs are often found in association. With the ankle joint, which is often at fault, the knee joint may sometimes show an ill-developed patellar tendons, blending with the sheath that connects the fibula with the distal femur. The foot which is usually in equinovarus position often has a very short and atrophic great toe.

Radiography

Radiographs at birth show in AP and lateral projections absence of tibia with equinovarus position of foot. In flexion deformity of knee the flexed fibula articulates with the lower end femur.

Treatment

Treatment is started immediately in the neonatal period with a toe-to-groin plaster cast for correction of equinovarus deformity, which is changed weekly for 2 months.[14] If electromyography is done, it will show usually normal activity in the tibialis anterior, extensor digitorum brevis and gastrocnemius muscles but diminished activity in the tibialis posterior, flexor digitorum longus and extensor hallucis longus. The last three tendons have a common fibrous insertion spread over the medial aspect of the foot having sometimes a connection with the tibialis anterior tendon. At 3 months of age telectomy is performed through a lateral incision. Tendo-Achilles is tenotomised and the lateral malleolus is pushed after necessary dissection, to centre of the dorsal surface of the calcaneus. The tibialis anterior tendon is transferred to cuboid, if necessary. The correction is maintained by repeated groin to toe casts upto the age of 6 months.

At that age the centralisation of the fibula is done at its upper end by a lateral approach. The fibrous distal expansion of the quadriceps tendon, which holds the fibular head nearer to femoral condyles terminates into an atrophied patellar tendon, which is attached to either of the hypoplastic femoral condyles. The fibular head is pushed to the inter-condylar notch and held in place with a thin Steinmann pin keeping the knee in maximum extension possible. The patellar tendon is transferred to the proximal fibular metaphysis or diaphysis. The residual equinovarus deformity of the foot is corrected in the same sitting by posteromedial soft tissue release and tendo-Achilles lengthening. The correction was maintained by groin to toe cast upto the age of one year. The patient was then allowed to walk with a long leg brace keeping the knee in maximum extension. The ankle is allowed to move freely.

The fibula gradually hypertrophies and takes the place of tibia. Good results are usually obtained with the attainment of satisfactory quadriceps power. Failure of this procedure will necessitate in arthrodesis of the knee and the fibulocalcaneal joints. Arthrodesis of the knee joint with distal amputation is recommended by some authors[13] in failed cases.

CONGENITAL LONGITUDINAL DEFICIENCY OF THE FIBULA

The diagnosis of this congenital deformity at birth is from a short leg with an outwardly twisted foot. The cause is failure of formation or arrest in the development of fibula, which takes place within 8 weeks of gestation. No teratogenic or hereditary factor has been found as the cause. This uncommon deformity occurs mostly unilaterally and is common in females.

Classification and Clinical Features

According to severity of the deficiency Achterman and Kalamchi[15] have classified the deformity into two different types. The type 1 A describes a hypoplastic short fibula with its upper epiphysis distal to the proximal epiphyseal cartilage of the tibia and the lower fibular epiphyseal cartilage is placed proximal to the ankle joint giving the foot slight valgus and equinus appearance. In the type 1B, there is partial deficiency of the fibula of its upper one-third or half (Fig. 14.3). The tibia is short and bowed anteromedially. The shortening is more with greater deficiency of the fibula. The femur is also shorter than the normal side. Type II describes absence of whole of fibula or only a distal vestigial fibrocartilaginous fibula is present. In the last type, the tibia is short with anteromedial bowing. The outer rays of the foot are absent along with absence of corresponding tarsal bones and the foot and ankle are in a position of equinovalgus (Fig. 14.4). Other associated findings are shortening of the femur, genu valgum with instability of the knee due to absence of either or both of the cruciate ligaments and hypoplastic high-riding and often subluxated patella. The ankle joint is in valgus with ball and socket appearance and is sometimes associated with coalition of the talus and calcaneum.

The deformity is often associated with abnormalities of the upper limb like shortening with syndactyly in fingers to total absence.

Predicted shortening of the lower limb in congenital longitudinal deficiency of the fibula was suggested by Choi and his associates,[16] classifying the deformities into three groups. They have classified the deformities into three groups according to the level of the foot of the affected limb at the distal third of the normal limb as Group I; the foot at the middle third of the normal limb as Group II and the position of the foot of the shorter limb at the upper third of the normal limb as Group III. In the group I with a

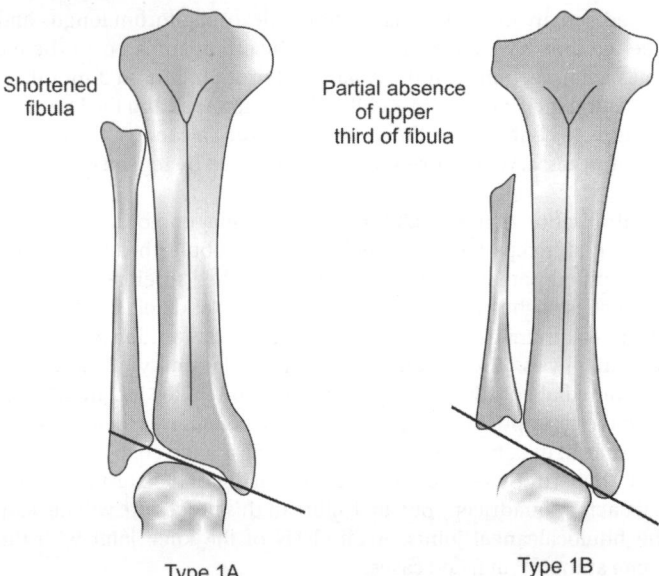

Fig. 14.3: Congenital longitudinal deficiency of the fibula-classified as type IA showing a hypoplastic short fibula and type IB denoting partial absence of the upper third of the fibula

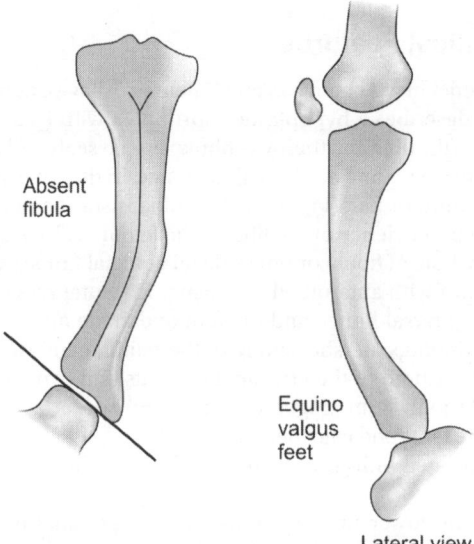

Fig. 14.4: Congenital longitudinal deficiency of the fibula-type II AP and lateral views showing absence of entire fibula with equinovalgus foot

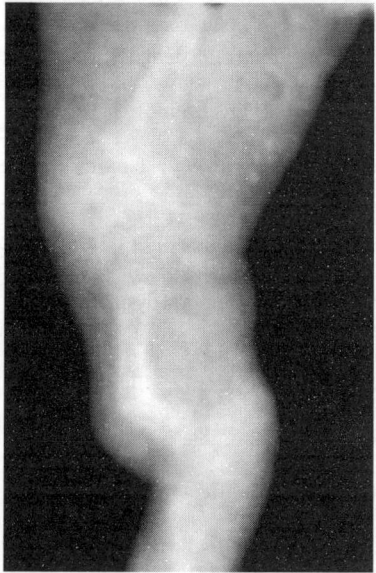 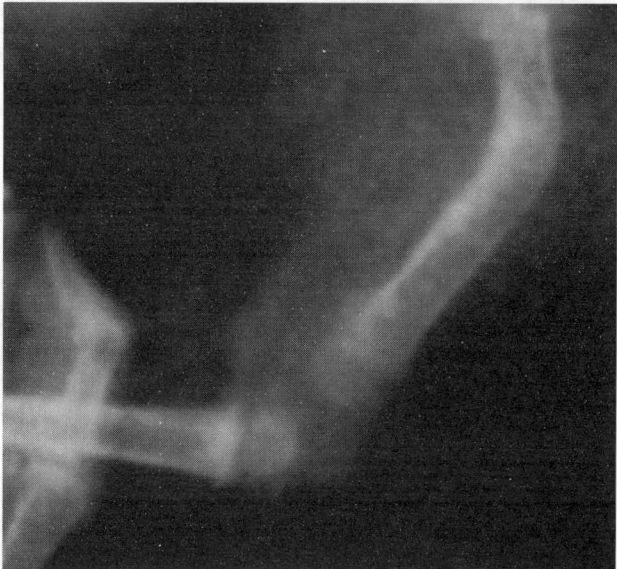

Fig. 14.5: Radiograph of a severe type II congenital longitudinal deficiency of the fibula with an anteriorly angulated short tibia

Fig. 14.6: The radiograph of the same patient as in Figure 14.5 at a later age with some straightening of the short tibia; instability in the ankle persists

shortening of 15 per cent the predicted limb length inequality at skeletal maturity was 0.5 to 12 cm. In group II of 16 to 25 per cent shortening the predicted limb length disparity was 12.5 to 23 cm and in group III with a shortening greater than 26 per cent the predicted limb length inequality was greater than 23 cm.

Treatment

The treatment of the condition is not that difficult in type I A. But in the management of type I B and type II (Figs 14.5 and 14.6) the severity of the deformity of the foot, instability of the ankle, mechanical axis deviation of the affected lower limb with valgus and instability at knee are to be considered to decide about multiple surgical procedures or amputation. Discussion will have to be made with the parents in the neonatal period regarding the ultimate outcome of gross shortening of the affected lower limb. The type I needs in the neonatal period stretching of the peronei and triceps surie and splinting the foot and ankle in an ankle-foot orthosis at night. The shortening which will develop later on will be corrected by shoe raise on the affected side when the child walks. If the disparity is pronounced the child may require epiphysiodesis of the contralateral proximal tibia and fibula at around the age of eight or nine years. For gross ankle valgus supramalleolar varus angulation osteotomy is recommended.

The management of the type II, variety (Fig. 14.5) is difficult because of a number of difficult problems of the condition described before, which may require multiple surgical procedures. In case of a hypoplastic and rigid foot with absence of two outer rays Syme's amputation is a better choice and should be performed before the child learns walking.

Shortening is corrected by tibial lengthening when the child attains 8 to 10 years of age. The methods adopted are either Ilizarov or Orthofix techniques.

REFERENCES

1. Torode IP, Gillespie R. Arteroposterior instability of the knee: A sign of congenital limb deficiency. J Pediatr Orthop 1983;3: 467-70.
2. Johansson E, Aparisi T. Missing cruciate ligament in congenital short femur. J Bone Jt. Surg 1983;65A:1109-1115.
3. Gillesspie R, Torode IP. Classification and management of congenital abnormalities of the femur. J Bone Jt Surg. 1983;65B:557-68.
4. Ring PA. Congenital short femur in simple femoral hypoplasia J Bone Joint Surg 1959;41B:73.
5. Hamanishi. Congenital short femur, clinical, genetic and epidemiological comparison of the naturally occurring condition with that caused by thalidomide J Bone Joint Surg (Br) 1980;62B:307-20.
6. Fixsen JA, Lloye-Roberts GC. The natural history and early treatment of proximal femoral dysplasia. J Bone Joint Sug 1974;56B.
7. Kalamchi A, Dawe RN. Congenital deficiency of the tibia. J Bone Jt Surg., 1978;60B:31.
8. Tuli SM, Verma BP. Congenital diastasis of the tibiofibular mortise. J Bone Jt Surg., 1972;54B:346.
9. Bose K. Congenital diastasis of the inferior tibiofibular joint. J Bone Jt. Surg, 1976;58A: 86.
10. Jones D, Barnes J, Lloyd-Roberts GC. Congenital aplasia and dysplasia of the tibia with intact fibula; classification and management. J Bone Jt. Surg., 1978;60B: 31.
11. Nutt JJ, Smith EE. Total congenital absence of the tibia. Am J. Roentgenol Radium Thera Nucl Med, 1941;46: 841-49.
12. Frantz CH, O'Rahilly R. Congenital skeletal limb deficiencies. J Bone Jt. Surg., 1961;43A:1202-24.
13. Kalamchi A, Dawe RV. Congenital deficiency of the tibia. J Bone Jt Surg, 1985;67B: 581.
14. Wehbe MA, Weinstein SL, Ponseti IV. Tibial agenesis. J Ped Orthop, 1981;1:395-99.
15. Achterman C, Kalamchi A. Congenital absence of fibula. J Bone Jt Surg 1979;61B:132.
16. Choi IH, Kumra SJ, Bowen JR. Amputation or limb-lengthening for partial or total absence of the fibula. J Bone Jt. Surg., 1990;72:1391.

Chapter 15

Proximal Femoral Focal Deficiency

Keywords: Congenital proximal femoral focal deficiency – caused by various noxious agents – classified into four varieties by Aitken and into five varieties by Amstutz – basic treatment is correction of instability of hip and limb length inequality.

Congenital focal deficiency of the proximal femur occurs infrequently and is associated with other developmental anomalies. The condition is a combination of upper femoral maldevelopment of variable degree and femoral shortening. Aitken[1] first introduced the term proximal femoral focal deficiency.

Various agents postulated as a cause of the condition include irradiation, anoxia, ischaemia, mechanical or thermal injury, bacterial toxins, viral infection, chemicals and hormones. But the use of thalidomide in the first trimester of pregnancy has been shown to be definite cause. Heredity is rarely a causative factor.

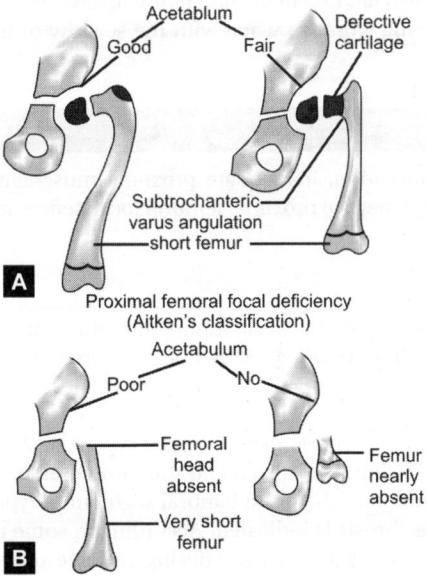

Figs 15.1A and B: Proximal femoral focal deficiency (Aitken's classification)

CLASSIFICATION

Aitkem[1], classified this disorder into four groups omitting the milder form with simple femoral shortening (Figs 15.1A and B). Amstutz[2] covered all the varieties and described five types.

Type 1

Congenital short femur with bowing, coxa vara, a normal acetabulum, delayed ossification of capital epiphysis and sclerosis of the medial femoral cortex.

Type 2

Short femur with subtrochanteric pseudoarthrosis where ossification will follow, associated with progressive coxa vara and a normal acetabulum.

Type 3

Short femur having a bulbous proximal end and delayed appearance of capital epiphysis in a dysplastic acetabulum.

Type 4

Upper end of femur is tapered and sclerosed with a tendency to proximal migration. The acetabulum becomes progressively dysplastic with a very delayed appearance of capital epiphysis.

Type 5

The proximal femur and acetabulum are absent. A small bony segment represents the distal femoral shaft.

The above varieties are often accompanied by absence of fibula with or without absence of outer two rays, kyphotic and/or hypoplastic or absent tibia. All the types except the fifth type will have development of the hip. The varus becomes extreme with time, being worse to worst with the severity of the types described above.

MANAGEMENT

Four basic problems, like instability of the hip, malrotation, inadequate proximal musculature and inequality of limb length need correction in the management of proximal femoral focal deficiency.

Instability of Hip

As the instability of hip varies with the development of the acetabulum and the union of the pseudoarthrosis, the question of development of the hip does not arise in type 5, where the remaining bone is fused with the bony pelvis and the musculature is developed through exercise and active weight bearing.

Various authors have corrected coxa vara by subtrochanteric osteotomy in Type 1 or 2. In some of the type 3 cases pseudoarthrosis is treated with excision of cartilage and the formed element from the attempt for bony fusion. In case of proximal migration of the distal femoral segment in type 2 or 3, exploration with excision and grafting of the pseudoarthrosis is indicated. According to some authors, bone formation at the pseudoarthrosis is stimulated mechanically by arthrodesing the knee and allowing weight bearing.

In the type 4, surgical exploration is unrewarding and the functional result is poor because of bony and muscular hypoplasia.

Malrotation and Inadequate Proximal Musculature

Correction of malrotation and inadequate proximal musculature helps in improving a fixed flexion and lateral rotation deformity of the hip, as is usually observed in these cases. Many authors advocate conversion of the leg to a single lever by fusion of the knee, which helps in reduction of the fixed flexion deformity.

Leg Length Inequality

There are four different ways of correcting leg length discrepancy. The help of an extension prosthesis is usually taken, where the foot is placed in equinus, and the type of prosthesis may either be below-knee or above-knee. Van Nes in 1950 performed rotation-plasty where the knee was arthrodesed after rotating the distal half of the limb through 180° bringing the ankle into a position where it functioned as a knee with the calf muscles acting as the quadriceps, the heel and the sole of the foot directing forward.

At present the choice of treatment is an early Syme's amputation as soon as the child learns walking and the process is further helped with an end-bearing prosthesis. However, the disproportionate growth in the thigh and the leg is put to some advantage by arthrodesis of the knee at a later age.

REFERENCES

1. Aitken GT. Proximal femoral focal deficiency - definition, classification and management in Proximal Femoral Focal Deficiency: A congenital Anomaly. National Academy of Sciences, 1969, 1.
2. Amstutz HC. The morphology, natural history and treatment of proximal femoral focal deficiency. In Aitken GT (Ed): Proximal Femoral Focal Deficiency; A Congenital Anomoly, National Academy of Sciences, 1969, 50.

Chapter 16

Congenital Coxa Vara

Keywords: Coxa vara – the diminished neck shaft angle of femur – three different varieties – clinically and radiographically detected – corrected by surgery – different types of osteotomies.

Coxa vara: The diminished neck shaft angle of femur, is a term derived from Latin words coxa means the hip joint and varus meaning angulation towards the midline of the body. The condition congenital coxa vara is found in infancy and childhood. A rare variety of it, is present at birth and is associated with congenital defects like short femur and other limb abnormalities; which appears to be related to environmental factors without any genetic involvement.[1] The other variety, an isolated congenital coxa vara, is often bilaterally symmetrical having some familial occurrences. The latter is more common than the first type and is detected when the child learns walking and hence is termed developmental or infantile coxa vara.[2] After histological studies Pylkkanen[3] suggested the cause of the defect as a disturbance of ossification and growth originating in the medial part of proximal femoral epiphyseal plate. A third variety has been reported which occurs due to a secondary congenital error associated with intrauterine affection of bone such as achondroplasia.[4]

PATHOLOGY

A progressively shortened lower limb due to progressive decrease in the neck shaft angle with a short neck of femur, having a defect at its medial part, forms the crux of the pathology. A vertically disposed epiphyseal plate is medial to the defect forming an inverted `V' and the metaphysis on the lateral side of the defect is osteoporotic with a triangular piece of bone separated from the inferior aspect of the neck, known as Fairbank's triangle, are the characteristics of the pathology[5] (Fig. 16.1). Microscopically, the defect is composed of cartilage and osteoid tissue.[6] The cartilage cells are arranged in an irregular columnar fashion and the ossification within it is irregular. The trabeculae in the adjoining osteoporotic metaphysis are atrophic containing occasionally large groups of cartilage cells. The head of the femur is normal.

If the deformity is left untreated the greater trochanter gradually extends upward towards the ilium; ultimately the trochanter goes much higher than the level of the head.

CLINICAL FINDINGS

Before the Child Learns Walking

From birth, the shortened lower extremity with free movements of the hip within the acetabulum raises suspicion of coxa vara, mostly associated with a short femur of type III.

Congenital Coxa Vara

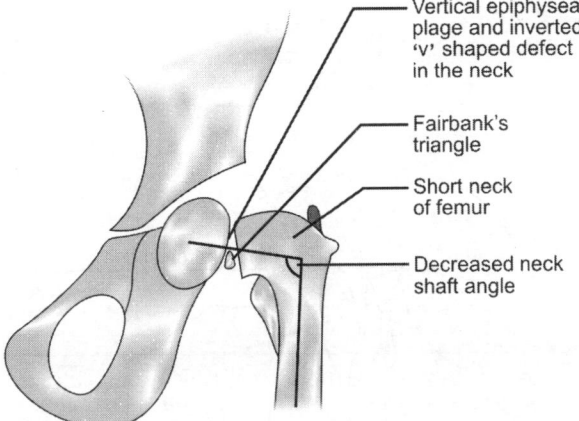

Fig. 16.1: Showing decreased neck shaft angle with short neck of femur having a vertically disposed epiphyseal plate and an inverted `V' shaped defect, the Fairbank's triangle being placed inferiorly

After the Child Learns Walking

A painless limp is the common complaint. In bilateral cases waddling gait is the presenting feature, caused by weak hip abductors. The hip movements are fairly normal without any telescoping sign. The greater trochanter lies above the Nelaton's line. The Trendelenburg's test is often positive because of weak abduction of the hip.

A Neglected Case in Adult Life

The waddling gait is pronounced. As the greater trochanter lies much above the head of the femur and often of bilateral occurrence, there is pain and stiffness of hip due to degenerative arthritis, which appear quite early. The abductors and flexors of hip gradually shorten and there is a progressive limitation of abduction and internal rotation.

RADIOGRAPHIC FEATURES

The characteristic finding in X-ray of a typical case of coxa vara are:
  i. The neck shaft angle of the femur is 90° or even less with retroversion of neck.
  ii. An oblique defect in the femoral neck extending upward toward the vertically disposed epiphyseal plate forming an inverted `V' with the latter.
  iii. The metaphysis is osteoporotic with a triangular fragment at its proximo-inferior part, placed in the inferior portion of the inverted `V' known as Fairbank's triangle.
  iv. The neck is short in length, its inferior border is concave forming a down-hanging lip and its superior border convex.
  v. The head, epiphyseal cartilage and the triangular fragment appear to be slipping downward as a unit.
  vi. The acetabulum is deformed as the head is radiolucent and lowly placed in it.
  vii. In neglected cases the greater trochanter is beak shaped goes up and almost touches the ilium.
  viii. Weinstein et al[7] in a retrospective review of 22 cases of congenital coxa vara introduced the Hilgenreiner epiphyseal (HE) angle as measured on the anteroposterior X-ray of the hips to determine the degree of coxa vara deformity. The HE angle is the angle between Hilgenreiner line on the horizontal axis and the line through the metaphyseal side of the femoral neck on the vertical axis—angle ABC (Fig. 16.2).

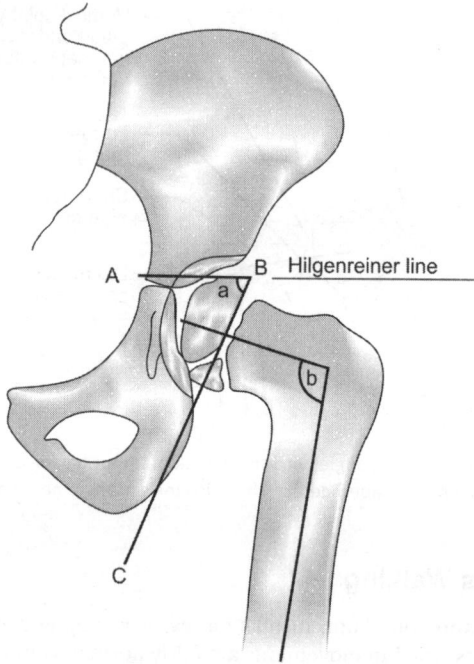

Fig. 16.2: Hilgenreiner's line and ∠ABC = Hilgenreiner's epiphyseal angle (a) and neck shaft angle shown as (b)

DIAGNOSIS

An isolated case of congenital coxa vara needs differentiation from coxa vara associated with congenital short femur of type III where the femoral shortening is the primary defect whereas coxa vara is predominant in the other. The femoral neck is not horizontal in the latter variety but retroverted and bent with irregular and mottled growth plate. Unlike the isolated coxa vara the other variety has marked thickening of the calcar in the femoral shaft with a hypoplastic or absent lesser trochanter. Although there is no incidence of familial occurrence in the congenital short femur variety, yet association with other limb abnormalities is not rare in it.

TREATMENT

The treatment is mainly operative correction of the deformity because:
  i. Conservative treatment is of little or no value.
  ii. If left untreated, there may develop a pseudoarthrosis at the defect and the head may lie widely separated from the neck.

So, the treatment should be started early before the age of eight years.[3] Operative restoration of proximal femur is indicated before the coxa vara and the limp are on the increase.[7] The aim of operative treatment is to realign the proximal femur; to prevent downward displacement of the head of the femur and supporting it from below by corrective osteotomy which makes the disposition of the vertical defect into a horizontal one. Various types of osteotomy had been advocated by different surgeons at different times.

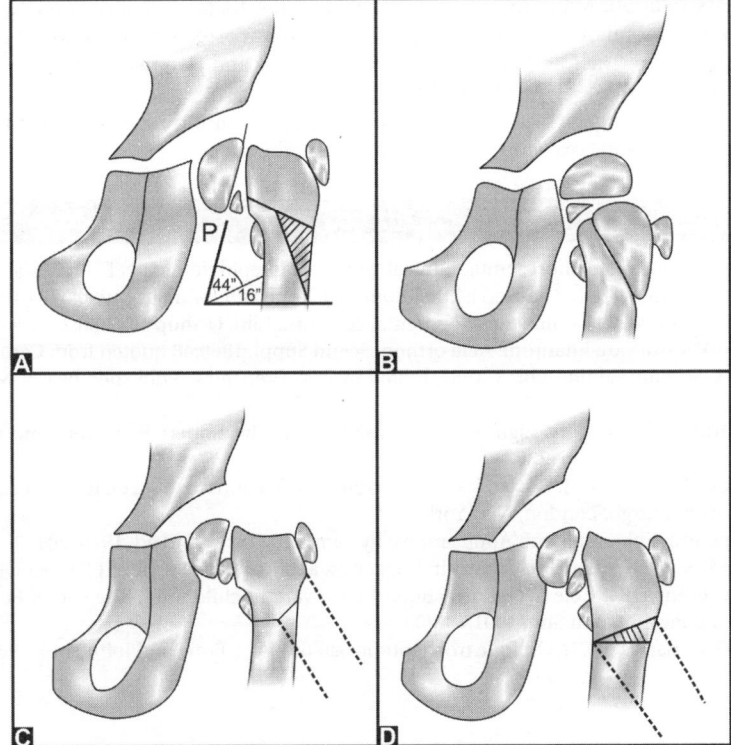

Figs 16.3A to D: (A) Plane in Pauwel's `Y' osteotomy with P representing plane of the growth plate, H being the horizontal line in the subtrochanteric femur, a 44 degree closing wedge osteotomy corrects the growth plate inclination to 16 degree; (B) After the osteotomy the femoral shaft fragment supports the triangular metaphyseal fragment and the displaced femoral head; (C) Showing abducted femoral shaft in stippled line following Dickson's geometric osteotomy; (D) Showing subtrochanteric valgus osteotomy with abducted femoral shaft in stippled line and the wedge in adjoining upper fragment, to be removed before aligning the fragments

Types of Osteotomies

i. Pauwels devised a Y-shaped intertrochanteric osteotomy where on closing the wedge component of the `Y' correction of the plane of the growth plate was achieved, while the stem component supported the epiphysis and the metaphyseal fragment[8] (Figs 16.3A and B).
ii. Dickson's geometric osteotomy (Fig. 16.3C) changes the femoral alignment, places the vertical defect into a horizontal position and abducted shaft of femur supports the head and also increases limb length.
iii. Subtrochanteric valgus osteotomy also serves the same purpose like the other two, where a small wedge is removed from the upper fragment before aligning the lower fragment into abduction (Fig. 16.3D). The osteotomies are fixed by various methods like pin-plate or blade plate fixation or by tension band wiring for Pauwels osteotomy.
iv. A different type of osteotomy was described by MacEwen and Shands[9] which corrects coxa vara as also retroversion of femoral neck. An oblique subtrochanteric osteotomy at an angle of 30 to 60° from anterosuperior to posteroinferior direction is made. Osteotomy made at 30 to long axis of shaft

produces less rotation. Maintaining contact between the fragments abduction of lower fragment produces internal rotation of the fragment as well, thereby corrects both coxa vara and retroversion of the neck of femur. The fragments are fixed with a screw and also two removable Steinmann pins fixed with pins-and-plaster type of cast.

As recurrence following correction of coxa vara is quite common regular follow-up is essential. A short femur associated with coxa vara needs operative lengthening.

REFERENCES

1. Hamanishi C. Congenital short femur, clinical genetic and epidemiological comparison of the nturally occurring condition with that caused by thalidomide J. Bone and Joint Surg 1980;62B (3): 307.
2. Fisher RI, Waskowitz WJ. Familial developmental coxa vara Clin. Orthop 1972;86:2.
3. Pylkkanen PV: Coxa vara infantum, Acta orthop. Scand Suppl. 1960;48 quoted from Campbell's operative orthopedics, Seventh Edition Vol. 3, 1987, Edited by A.K. Crenshow, Published by C.V. Mosby Company, 2750.
4. Mercer's Orthopedic Surgery Eighth Edition 1983, Edited by Robert B. Duthie and George Bentley. Published by Edward Arnold, 238.
5. Wynne - Davis R, Fairbank TJ. Fairbank's Atlas of General Affections of the skeleton, 2nd ed. 1976, Churchill Livingstone: Edinburgh, London, New York.
6. Orthopedics, Principles and their Applications: by Samuel L. Turek, 3rd ed, 1978, 284.
7. Weinstein JN, Kuo KN Millar EA. Congenital coxa vara a retrospective review, J Pediatr Orthop 1984;4:70.
8. Cordes S, Dickens DRV, Cole WG. Correction of coxa vara in childhood: The use of Pauwels' Y-shaped osteotomy, J Bone and Joint Surg 1991;73B(1).
9. MacEwen GD, Shands AD, Jr. Oblique trochanteric osteotomy, J. Bone and Joint Surg. 1967;49-A, 345.

Chapter 17

Foetal Development and Natural History of Lower Limb Rotation

Keywords: The version – the normal twisting or rotation of a long bone on its anatomic longitudinal axis occurring during gestation - reverses completely in the neonatal period – an increase or decrease or rotation is termed as antetorsion, which is a deformity.

The neonatal period is the turning point when the rotation or version of the femur and tibia during the gestation reverses completely. Version is the normal twisting of a long bone on its anatomic longitudinal axis. Foetal development of the limbs and their rotation need a short description in order to understand clearly the rotation of the limbs. During the fourth to fifth week of gestation, a bud develops on the ventrolateral body wall, which is the limb bud. The end of this bud flattens to form a plate. The digits are formed from the condensation of mesenchyme of this plate and dissolution of tissues between the rays. The toes are formed at around 8th week of gestation and the feet are placed in a position apposed to each other, known as 'praying feet' position. The great toes thus are placed upwards taking a pre-axial position. With further growth of the foetus the lower limbs rotate medially and the feet assume plantigrade position. The thumbs in the hands follow the same. Now rotation takes place in the limb bud; the femur rotating laterally and the tibia medially. The femoral anteversion is 35° at birth, which gradually decreases with age reaching a figure of 8° in an adult male and 14° in a female. The tibiofibular version is interestingly lateral in the gestational period, gradually decreasing towards full-term and in the newborn the transmalleolar axis/plane is medially placed with reference to the transcondylar axis/plane. The value of tibial version, on an average, is 2 to 4° lateral at birth and 10 to 20° lateral in the adult. I would like to make out the difference between the term version and torsion.

VERSION

Version is the normal twisting of a long bone on its anatomic longitudinal axis as said earlier. When this twisting or rotation is increased or decreased giving a measurement greater or lesser than two standard deviation (SD) of the mean, the rotational alignment is termed as antetorsion, which is a deformity.

To describe the torsional defects in a long bone like femur and tibia, the inclination or the angle between the axis or plane of the femoral or tibial condyles with the axis of the femoral neck or the transmalleolar axis is measured.

The tibiofibular torsion in the growing foetus was studied by Badelon[1] and his associates from the foetal period until birth and showed an increased lateral tibiofibular torsion in the early foetal life gradually changing in the newborn to medial tibiofibular torsion. After birth tibia rotates laterally.

Normally acetabular anteversion is − 2 to 16° (mean 7°)[2] and remains almost constant during the first-half of gestation and during childhood. There is a reciprocal relationship between the degree of acetabular anteversion and that of femoral anteversion.

REFERENCES

1. Badelon O, Bensahel H, Folinais D, Lessale B. Tibiofibular torsion from the foetal period until birth. J Pediatr Orthop 1989;9:169.
2. Browning WH, RosenKrantz H, Tarquinio T. Computed Tomography in congenital hip dislocation. The role of acetabular anteversion. J Bone Jt Surg 1982;64A: 27.

Chapter 18

Postural and Congenital Deformities of the Foot and Ankle

Keywords: Deformities of foot and ankle at birth – caused by posture of the baby in the uterus or by some congenital intrinsic defect or a spinal defect like myelomeningocele – the metatarsus or the foot as a whole or the toes are involved in the deformities.

Deformities of the foot and the ankle at birth may be caused by lie or posture of the baby in the uterus or due to some congenital intrinsic defect or from some paralytic affection due to a spinal defect like myelomeningocele. The postural defects are easily corrected as the baby is free from its uterine position. Only a few requires some manipulation or splintage for correction. The congenital deformities need correction primarily by plastering or splintage; failing which operative treatment is the only answer.

The postural defects are evident in almost all the parts of the body from foot upwards like metatarsus adductus, metatarsus primus varus, calcaneovalgus, pes plano valgus, pes equino valgus, medial or lateral tibiofibular torsion, genu recurvatum, lateral rotation contracture of the hip, pelvic obliquity with adduction contracture of one hip and abduction contracture of the opposite hip. These deformities may occur alone or in combination. The spine may be affected as postural infantile scoliosis and the head and neck may show postural torticollis and plagiocephaly. These deformities usually do not require active treatment in the neonatal period except in some severe form which may require repeated passive stretching and rarely plastering. Maintenance of correction will be achieved by passive stretching while the baby is awake and splintage at night for 3 to 4 weeks.

METATARSUS ADDUCTUS VERSUS CONGENITAL METATARSUS VARUS

The appearance of the deformed foot is almost same in both the conditions with adduction of forefoot at the tarso-metatarsal joints having an extra skin crease on the medial plantar aspect of the foot in the congenital variety.

Metatarsus Adductus

This is a forefoot adduction deformity maintaining hindfoot neutrality. The abductor hallucis muscle is taut. There is frequent association of developmental hip dysplasia with this deformity. The treatment when required is repeated passive stretching exercises.

Congenital Metatarsus Varus

The deformity shows forefoot adduction and inversion at the tarso-metatarsal joints, which are often due to subluxation. A crease is present on the medial plantar aspect of foot. The condition at birth needs only passive stretching for correction. If not treated, the deformity increases in severity with convexity of the lateral border of the foot and prominence of the base of the 5th metatarsal. The abductor hallucis muscle becomes taut. Repeated manipulation and plastering are necessary for the correction of the severe deformity.

CONGENITAL TALIPES CALCANEOVALGUS

The deformity of the foot which an orthopaedic surgeon is very often asked to see in the neonatal period is congenital talipes calcaneovalgus. The sole of the foot looks outwards and upwards and the foot is dorsiflexed at the ankle with eversion and abduction at the subtalar and midtarsal joints. The deformity is usually mild when the foot is easily inverted and adducted by passive manipulation. The difficulty in passive correction is due to contracted dorsiflexors of the ankle and the peroneus brevis muscle. The deformed feet are graded mild, moderate and severe according to the range of passive correction upto beyond neutral, to neutral and no change. Sometimes these deformities are associated with dysplasia of the hip with subluxation. Spinabifida and other vertebral column defects are often associated. Angulation of the tibia and the fibula towards posteromedial side is often found with this deformity.

Treatment of mild and moderate varieties is by manipulation and stretching of contracted dorsal and lateral structures turning foot towards reverse direction of plantar flexion and inversion. Manipulation is done several times a day, twenty to thirty time on each occasion. Only the severe variety needs correction in a plaster cast, manipulating the plastered foot to plantar flexion when the plaster sets. One or two plastering at two or three weeks' interval are necessary to achieve full correction.

The sequal of this deformity is development of planovalgus deformity of foot in a young infant with an obliquely placed talus in the radiograph.

CONGENITAL CONVEX PES VALGUS AT BIRTH

The condition was first described by Henken[1] in 1914. Lamy and Weiseman[2] suggested the name congenital convex pes valgus. The term congenital convex pes valgus was used by Herndon and Heymen[3] in preference to congenital vertical talus as this nomenclature denotes the clinical deformity. This is a rare condition, often difficult to diagnose, when first examined after birth. The deformity appears quite similar to congenital talipes calcaneovalgus and plantar flexed talus seen in paralytic or spastic flat foot. Differentiation is often a problem. The presenting features are convex sole in flat foot with the toes looking upwards and the head of the talus is felt as a bony prominence on the plantar aspect of the foot giving a rocker-bottom appearance of the foot.

Etiology

The cause of this deformity is not known. An arrest of prenatal development of feet at around 8 weeks causing a stoppage of dorsiflexion, which normally occurs, has been incriminated as the cause. Dorsolateral displacement of the talocalcanenavicular and calcaneocuboid joints *in utero* causes the deformity. Familial incidence of the condition has been observed but no hereditary predisposition was detected. The author could diagnose six feet of isolated congenital vertical talus in five patients among thirty feet in twenty-eight babies with planovalgus feet in a study carried out between 1975 and 1981.[4]

Classification

The deformity in congenital convex pes valgus may occur as a primary one in the form of an isolated deformity or may be in association with other musculoskeletal deformitis like congenital dislocation of hip, congenital dislocation of knee, contralateral talipes equinovarus or calcaneovalgus deformity or as one of the numerous anomalies in trisomy 13 to 15 or 18.

The condition may happen secondary to neuromuscular disorders like myelomeningocele, lumbosacral agenesis, caudal regression syndrome or arthrogryposis multiplex congenita.

Pathology

A typical case of vertical talus shows the following characteristics:
a. Plantar displacement of the head of the talus with the navicular displaced dorsally and articulating with the neck of the talus, locking the latter in a vertical position.
b. Posterior displacement of the calcaneus in relation to the talus with a deficiency in the anterior support of the head of the talus.
c. Abduction and valgus of the forefoot—produced as a result of an increase in length of the medial side of the foot because of relative forward displacement of the talus on the calcaneum. The cuboid is slightly dorsally displaced.
d. The capsules and ligaments on the dorsolateral aspect of the talonavicular and calcaneocuboid joints are contracted.
e. Equinus of calcaneum with contracture of tendo-calcaneus, posterior capsule of the ankle and the subtalar joints.
f. Contracture of the peronei, extensor hallucis longus, extensor digitorum longus and the tibialis anterior.

Clinical Features

Rigid forefoot and midfoot with fixed abduction, dorsiflexion and eversion in a flat and valgus foot, resisting passive plantar flexion and inversion with the heel in equinus and valgus giving the foot a rocker-bottom appearance is the characteristic of the deformity. The prominent head of the talus on the plantar and medial aspect and the contracted tendons and muscles on the dorso-lateral aspect of the foot are easily palpable with the skin on it showing characteristic folds. Passive plantar flexion and inversion of the foot will not correct the deformity.

Radiographic Investigations

The dorsiplantar view shows lateral deviation of the forefoot with increase in talocalcaneal angel. The lateral view denotes plantar flexed calcaneum and its long axis passes plantar to cuboid; vertically displaced talus, whose axis is almost in a line with the vertical axis of tibia, posterior to cuboid; the cuboid (which casts shadow between birth and three weeks) is malaligned and the longitudinal axis of the first metatarsal points dorsal to talus denoting dorsally displaced radiologically uncast navicular. On passive plantar flexion of the foot, the vertical position of the talus remains unchanged.

The patients with congenital vertical talus should be investigated for AP and lateral views of the entire spine or ultrasonography to exclude vertebral anomalies like spinabifida, diastematomyelia, sacral agenesis and intraspinal lipoma or hydromyelia.

Differential Diagnosis

That congenital vertical talus deformity has got distinct difference from obliquely placed talus arising out of either flexible or paralytic pes planovalgus, is clear from both in the clinical and radiological findings. Passive plantar flexion of the deformity causes unchanged radiological appearance of vertical disposition of talus in congenital vertical talus deformity unlike that in the other two varieties with obliquely placed talus, where the deformity is corrected on passive plantar flexion of foot. Tarsal qualition causing spastic flat foot may mimic vertical talus deformity but ultrasonography of the tarsal bones clears the picture.

Treatment

In the neonatal period, the attempt to correct the deformity is by serial weekly change of plaster. Correction when obtained is maintained by splints. Failures are corrected at a later age by surgery.

NEONATAL DEFORMITIES OF THE TOES

Congenital Hallux Varus

In this condition, the great toe is deviated medially at the metatarsophalangeal joint and the first metatarsal is often short. The first metatarsophalangeal joint is sometimes found subluxated. The condition may occur as a primary deformity from contraction of fibrous tissues or may be part of a generalised bone dysplasia like diastrophic dwarfism. Sometimes the hallux is duplicated. No treatment is necessary in the neonatal period. Surgical correction is recommended between 6 and 12 months of age of baby because the deformity is often very rigid.

Metatarsus Primus Varus

In this condition, the great toe is deviated medially from the metatarsophalangeal joint creating a wide gap between the great and the second toes. The cause is tightness of the abductor hallucis muscle. Passive stretching exercise and splinting at night are required generally for the correction in the neonatal period. In severe cases manipulation and plastering may be necessary for a number of times and the condition may persist till the child learns walking.

Syndactyly

Failure of separation of adjoining fingers in embryonic life causes this deformity. The deformity may be partial or compete and usually is asymptomatic. Attempt at separation of toes may invite post-treatment problems. Hence, the condition is best left alone.

Symphalangism

This condition is also caused by failure of separation of adjoining fingers in embryonic life and arises due to fusion of two or three phalanges of a digit. This hereditary malformation of autosomal dominant trait is detected clinically at birth and is more common among Caucasians; occurs occasionally in Asians and rare among Blacks.

Any of the interphalangeal joints of one or more fingers or toes are affected. A short or absent middle phalanx is often an accompaniment. Syndactyly is often associated.

The affected finger or toe is stiff with the absence of active or passive motion in the affected joints. Periarticular soft tissues are atrophic and the volar or dorsal creases overlying the fused interphalangeal joints are absent. The condition does not pose much problem in the toes as it does in the hands.

The radiological detection of the deformity is not possible after birth because of the presence of cartilage. No treatment is done in the neonatal period. Modern treatment of callotasis with the help of various fixators is undertaken in the adolescent period.

Lobster Claw or Cleft Foot Deformity

This rare deformity where absence of the central two or three rays of the foot is often combined with similar deformity in the hand. Often inherited as an autosomal dominant and bilateral in nature, this malformation is associated frequently with cleft lip and palate. Sometimes the deformity is unilateral, when it is not hereditary.

Treatment, although is not very satisfactory, may be of some use to the patient. The first and fifth metatarsals are osteotomised at their bases and approximation of their distal end is done producing a sort of partial syndactyly. No treatment is necessary in the neonatal period.

Polydactyly or Supernumerary Digits

These may be on the medial side of the big toe, i.e. pre-axial or on the lateral side of the little toe or post-axial. Rarely they may be central. The condition is of autosomal dominant trait and is often associated with polydactyly of the hand. The deformities may be part of some syndrome like Ellis-van Creveld or Jeune's infantile thoracic dystrophy or Meckle syndrome. Longitudinal deficiency of tibia may also be associated.

Treatment is cosmetic, without disturbing growth. No treatment is necessary in the neonatal period. The time of excision of accessory toe is just before one year, before the child learns walking and the foot is big enough. Repair of capsule of the metatarsophalangeal joints should be thorough to prevent subluxation.

Macrodactyly

Excessive growth of toe may involve one or more toes. This condition may be true gigantism where all the tissues are hypertrophied, differing from false gigantism where one tissue is primarily involved. True gigantism may be primary condition when the etiology is unknown or the idiopathic variety and a secondary affection to neurofibromatosis or hemihypertrophy. In false gigantism the bone is hypertrophied as in Ollier's disease or melorheostosis, involvement of blood vessels as in Klippel-Trenaunay syndrome or haemangiomatosis causing hypertrophied digit or neurofibromatosis or lipomatosis or congenital lymphoedema causing gigantism.

The condition may be part of a syndrome like Proteus syndrome where a variety of hamartomatous conditions coexist causing muscle haemangioma, hemihypertrophy with hypertrophied digits and deformities specially valgus of the hips, the knees and the ankles with or without dislocation.

This condition needs no treatment in the neonatal period. The treatment is either by growth arrest of the metatarsal or phalanx or by total or partial excision of hypertrophied tissues.

REFERENCES

1. Henken R. Contribution a l'etude des formes osseuses du pied valgus congenital. Theses de Lyon, 1914.
2. Lamy L, Weissman L. Congential convex pes valgus, J Bone Joint Surg 1939;21:79.
3. Herndon CH, Heyman CH. Problems in the recognition and treatment of congenital convex pes valgus, J Bone Joint Surg 1939;45A:413.
4. De Mazumder N. Problems in the diagnosis of congenital convex pes valgus at birth. J. Vivekananda Institute of Med. Sciences 1979.p.2.

Chapter 19

Club Foot

Keywords: Club foot – history – etiology – morbid anatomy – incidence – clinical and radiographic features – conservative and operative treatment in the neonatal period.

The generic term talipes is derived from the Latin words talus means ankle and pes means foot. The term was first proposed by Little[1] in 1839 and was used to describe all foot deformities. To designate the specific forms of these deformities, Little used the terms varus, valgus and equinus. As a typical talipes equinovarus deformity, with equinus and varus deformities of the foot, looks like a club, the deformity is known as club foot.

CLUB FOOT

History

The history of club foot dates back to the days of ancient Egyptians. Wall paintings of their tombs depicted the club foot deformity. Aztecs in Mexico treated club foot deformity with splints made of cactus leaves. That most of the club feet are corrected and that these are caused mechanically was first proposed by Hippocrates[2] around 300 BC. He also emphasized on an early start of the treatment with repeated gentle stretching before the deformity in the bones became well-established. Strong bandages were used during manipulative correction, and shoes for the maintenance of correction.

Etiology

Although the cause of the club foot is unknown, yet the occurrence of most of the congenital idiopathic club feet is attributed to an abnormality in foetal environment, arresting embryonic development at a crucial stage; hereditary predisposition is probably an added factor in many cases. Many authors agree that the deformity probably results from a combination of multifactorial polygenic predisposition and some obscure intrauterine environmental factor. The effect of hereditary factor in the production of club foot was raised among others like Wynne-Davies[3] and Palmar[4] who showed an increased incidence of club foot among relatives of affected children. Contradictory genetic mechanisms have been proposed to explain the mode of inheritance, which remain unclear even today (Table 19.1).

The theory of mechanical compression in the uterus was first suggested by Hippocrates.[2] The opponents of this theory put forward an absence of increased incidence of club foot among twins, large babies, first born children, and in foetus developing in a relatively small roomed uterus. The protagonists like Denis Browne[5] maintained as a cause, a sudden increase in intrauterine pressure at a certain period of development of the foetus.

Heuter and von Volkmann[6] were the proponents of the idea of arrest of foetal development early in embryonic life in the etiology of congenital club foot, which was opposed by Bassel Hagen[7] but supported by Bohm.[8] However, no intrauterine noxious agent could be found influencing intrauterine environment and foetal development.

A germ plasm defect of the head of the talus was attributed to the etiology by Walsingham and Hughes[9] and later on Irani and Sherman.[10] The last named authors were of opinion that the defect must take place before the talus and tarsal joints develop at 6th week of intrauterine life. Antagonists of this theory attribute this abnormality of the talus to secondary adaptive changes. Duraiswamy injected insulin in the chick embryo and produced club foot deformity.

Issacs et al[11] opined after histochemical and electron microscopic studies on 60 club feet of patients aged five years and below that a neurogenic factor may be predominant as a cause. They considered idiopathic club foot as a resistant form of arthrogryposis multiplex congenita and that the legs in both are almost indistinguishable. Ionasecu and associates[12] showed muscle fibrosis in gastroenemius muscles as the cause. Others however, did not find any such abnormality.

A Victoria Diaz[13] studying[59] embryonic feet suggested distal tibial and fibular growth spurts affecting the position of the embryonic feet and the movements of the talus and the calcaneum. In the first stage—the fibular phase, the downwardly pushed calcaneum makes the foot assume an equinovarus position, corrected in the next tibial phase, when the talus is pushed down. An arrest of foetal growth after the fibular phase will produce a club foot. No definite neuromuscular defect has been incriminated as a cause of club foot, even on histochemical analysis.

The etiological factors (the causes) and their effects are given in the Table 19.1.

Morbid Anatomy

The first classical account on the pathologic anatomy of club foot was given by Scarpa[14] in 1803. He described congenital dislocation of the astragalo-calcaneo-scaphoid complex as the prime defect in a club foot. Adams[15] observed medial deviation of the head and neck of the talus in a club foot, which he thought, had developed as a secondary adaptive change and not a primary defect. Brockman[16] described the morbid anatomy as a congenital atresia of the astragalo-calcaneoscaphoid joint. Dillwyn Evans[17] stated a medial deviation of the foot at the midtarsal joint causing the deformity along with an elongation

Table 19.1: Etiology of club foot

Cause	Effect
Abnormality in foetal environment	Arresting embryonic development at a crucial stage
Mechanical compression in the uterus due to sudden increase in intrauterine pressure at a certain period of development of foetus	Making a hindrance to normal growth of the foetal parts
Arrest of foetal development early in embryonic life	Normal development of foetal parts comes into jeopardy
Germ plasm defect of the head of the talus at the 6th week of intrauterine life	Abnormal angle of the talar head and neck with diminished size of the head and neck.
Arrest of foetal growth after fibular phase (first to occur before tibial phase)	The position of foot in the equinovarus position due to fibular phase remains—causing club foot
Hereditary factor	Incresed incidence of club foot among relative of affected children
Multifactorial polygenic predisposition (the mode of inheritance is not simple).	Causing wide range of clinical variety

of the lateral column of the foot, whereas Attenborough[18] believed the primary defect as a plantar flexed talus. Goldner[19] along with others believed an increased lateral rotation of the talus in the ankle mortise.

A classical club foot deformity shows equinus, adduction and inversion in both the hindfoot and forefoot along with cavus in midfoot in some of the deformities. In the hindfoot, the head and the neck of the talus look downward and medially with the head assuming a wedge shaped appearance in a severe deformity. The anterior part of the superior articular surface of the talus is broader than the posterior part.[20] The calcaneum is inverted. McKay[21] opines that the calcaneum is malrotated in the transverse plane its posterior tuberosity going upwards and laterally. The navicular is displaced medial to the head of the talus, often positioned below the medial malleolus, separated from it by a fibrocartilaginous disc.[22] The cuboid moves with the calcaneum with which it is firmly articulated but occasionally is displaced medially from its articulation with the anterior process of calcaneum.[23,24] The forefoot and midfoot are adducted and plantar flexed. The forefoot is inverted too. The soft tissues on the plantar, medial and posterior aspects of the deformed foot including the ligaments, muscles and tendons are contracted. There are deep skin creases on the plantar and medial aspects and just above the heel. The great toe is often short and the foot size is smaller than the normal side due to the presence of smaller sized tarsal bones. Calf muscles are often atrophied. Association of tibia vara and internal tibial torsion with club foot has been over emphasised. The basic defect is in the foot with adaptive changes in the leg. Slight external rotation of ankle, which is present normally, is increased in club foot. Accessary attachment of tendons found in club foot has been hypothetised as secondary to bony deformity. Turco[25] opines that the magnitude of the deformity depends upon the degree of bony displacement, whereas rigidity of soft tissue contractures on the postero-medial part of foot is responsible for the resistance to treatment. Torsion of tibia associated with club foot has been thought to be of different types by different authors. While external tibial torsion was described by Lloyd Roberts et al[26,27] internal tibial torsion was supported by Brockman,[16] Kite[28] and Salter.[29] Wynne Davies,[30] Herold and Marcovich[31] found no significant degree of torsion.

Incidence

The deformity occurs in about one per 1000 live births, according to studies from Britain and Scandinavia. In Orientals, the incidence is about half that in Europeans; in Polynesians the disorder occurs about six times more as among Maori babies, but fortunately corrected mostly by manipulation as a domiciliary treatment. Prevalence of club foot is seen in Mexico, in the middle East and in countries on the Mediterranean coast of North Africa.

A child born to a family where one sibling is already suffering from the deformity is more likely to be affected by it than the normal population. A boy born to a family, having an affected girl among its members, is about twenty times more likely to suffer from the defect. Children of an affected mother are prone to suffer from club foot. Studies on twins reveal that concordance is more common in homozygous than in heterozygous twins.

Boys are affected twice as commonly as the girls. About half the cases are bilateral with a tendency towards involvement of right side more than the left.

Clinical Features

The affected foot has had all the components of the deformity—adduction, varus and equinus in both the forefoot and the hindfoot, with medial deviation of the midfoot giving the lateral border of the foot a roundish appearance (Fig. 19.1). The sole of the foot looks medially with the medial border of the foot, in a severe deformity, lying almost vertically above the lateral border (Fig. 19.2). The heel is in varus and often tucked up. Skin creases are prominent on the medial and plantar surfaces of the foot and just above the heel (Fig. 19.3). The calf muscles are atrophied and the great toe is occasionally small (Fig. 19.4). Pandey and Pandey[32] classified club foot into mild, moderate, severe and very severe on the basis

Club Foot

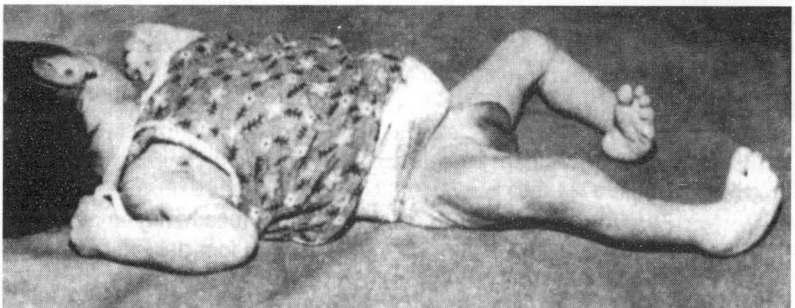

Fig. 19.1: Bilateral club foot deformity—classical variety

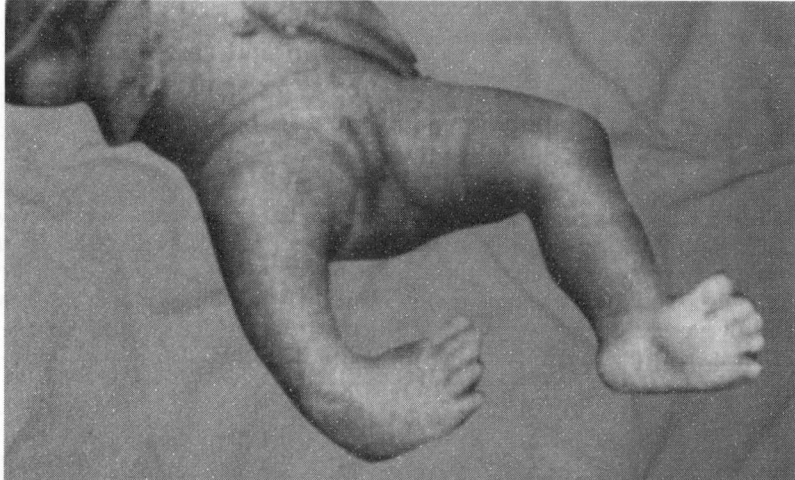

Fig. 19.2: Severe type of club foot deformity of right foot having the sole directed medially and the medial border of the foot lying almost vertically above the lateral border

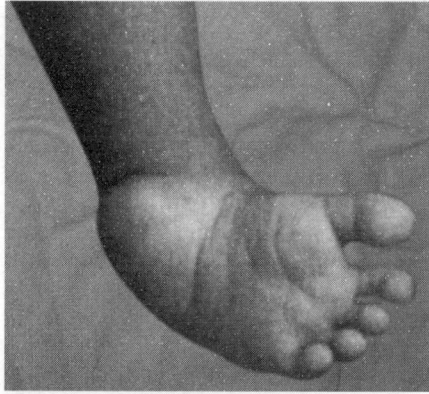

Fig. 19.3: Skin creases being prominent in this club foot

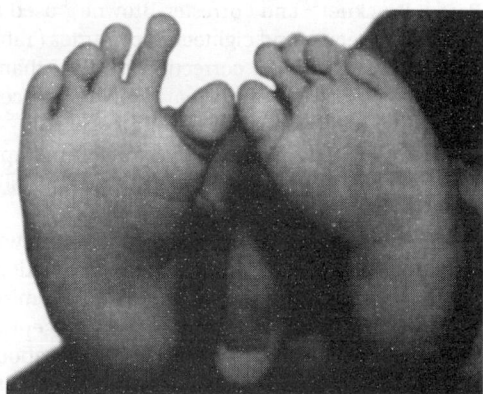

Fig. 19.4: The great toes being small in these bilateral club foot deformities

of skin condition, attitude of foot, stretchability of deformity, condition of heel and calf, feel of the calf and response to treatment. Club foot is often associated with supramalleolar lateral rotation of tibia as mentioned earlier. Internal torsion of tibia, as an associated deformity, is not very frequent according to the present author.

Deformities are classified into supple and rigid varieties according to their compliance to passive correction. A supple foot can be corrected to normal, whereas a rigid foot resists passive stretching.[33,34] Harrold and Walker[35] classified the deformity as mild or grade 1, if the deformed foot could be passively corrected to neutral or beyond the neutral position. Resistance to the above and the persistence of fixed equinus and varus to 20° or less was denoted as moderate or grade 2. The disorder with a fixed deformity of equinus and varus above 20° was considered severe or grade 3. On the basis of foot print analysis deformed feet were classified as mild, moderate or severe.[36] Catterall classified club feet as resolving, tendon contracture and joint contracture.[37]

According to Turco,[25] rigid feet are those small feet with markedly inverted and plantar flexed heels with or without a deep cleft above the heel or in the plantar surface, not responding to several months of manipulation and cast treatment. He concurs with McCaulay[38] that a deformed foot is considered as resistant when it does not show evidence of improvement with manipulations and presents both clinically and radiologically the persistence of equinovarus deformity.

Radiographic Features

Like a normal foot, a club foot at birth shows only two tarsal bones—the talus and the calcaneum, and the metatarsals. The cuboid makes its appearance at around 0 to 3 weeks; and the nucleus of navicular appears not before the third year. Therefore, in the neonatal period a club foot deformity is best assessed clinically. It is well known that the lateral view in a club foot, where the foot remains in an equinus position, mimics lateral X-ray of a normal foot in equinus. Hence the importance of lateral view of dorsiflexed foot,[25] which is difficult to obtain in a club foot. However, AP X-ray is informative in denoting inverted calcaneum under the talus in a club foot by showing a narrow talo-calcaneal angle.

Treatment

Various types of treatment have been advocated for congenital idiopathic club foot since the days of Hippocrates. Repeated gentle stretching and bandaging immediately after birth, as practised by Hippocrates[2] around 300 BC was followed till the time of Fabricius Hildamus,[39] who first used a mechanical appliance, like a boot hinged with a plate, for gradual correction of club foot. Arcaeus,[40] Pare,[41] Bruckner[42] and Forrester-Browne[43] used mechanical contrivances for the treatment of club foot in the seventeenth and eighteenth centuries (Table 19.2).

The use of gradual correction by a mechanical device like a shoe attached to a turnbuckle was practised by Scarpa[14] in the early nineteenth century. Various types of splints were used by Adams,[15] Lorenz,[44] Judson[45] and Dalton.[46]

Thomas[47] believed in applying forcible manipulation for the correction of club foot by using a wrench. Denis Browne.[48] used forcible manipulation followed by using his own splint for the maintenance of correction.

The treatment of club foot took a new turn with the use of plaster of Paris. Guerin[49] first used plaster for the correction of deformity after manipulation. Whitman,[50] Jones and Lovett[51] and Brockman[16] used adhesive strapping for the correction of deformity.

Most of the authors of the twentieth century are proponents of gentle manipulative correction immediately after birth as Apley[52] opined about better stretching of ligaments and capsules on the medial side of the deformed foot before two months of age. Chacko and Mathew[53] remarked that forcible manipulation causes uncontrolled tears in the ligaments and capsules on the medial side of the deformed foot producing stiffness. Many years ago Kite[54] practised gradual correction of components of deformity

Club Foot

Table 19.2: The trend and the type of conservative treatment of club foot

Type of treatment	The person introduced the treatment	The time of introduction
Repeated gentle stretching and bandaging immediately after birth	Hippocrates, Graham Apley	Around 300 BC
	Chacko and Mathews	1976
Mechanical appliance like a boot hinged with a plate was used for gradual correction	Fabricins Hildamus	1646
	Areaeus	1658
	Pare	1665
	Scarpa	1818
Splints used for correction	Adams	1873
	Loreuz	1884
	Judson	1892
Forcible manipulation for correction using mechanical contrivances	Bruckner	1796
	Thomas	1886
	Denis Browne	1934
First use of plaster of Paris to hold the correction after manipulation	Guerin	1838
Use of adhesive strapping for the correction	Whitman	1896
	Jones and Lovett	1929
	Brockman	1930
Serial wedge plastering	Kite	1930
Use of a forefoot abduction device with a turnbuckle for gradual correction	De Mazumdar	1978
Correction of all the components of the deformity in the same sitting	Turco	1981

by wedge plastering. Shaw[55] reviewed three different methods: (i) gentle stretching with Jones strapping, (ii) manipulation and serial plastering and (iii) use of Denis Browne splint as a corrective measure and found the first one producing the best result.

A forefoot abduction device with a turn-buckle (Fig. 19.5) is used by De Mazumder[33,34] for gradual dynamic correction of deformity except the equinus at ankle, the instrument being incorporated under the sole of the foot on the above knee plaster maintaining a wedge at the midtarsal region on the outer side of the deformed foot, the side of placement of turn-buckle. The plaster controlling hindfoot extends from midtarsal joint to above knee and the other controlling forefoot and midfoot extends from toes to midtarsal joint being kept closer at the dorsomedial part by incorporating a small spring within the plaster (Figs 19.6A to C). The spring prevents the forefoot part of the plaster to slip off. The heel is manipulated into valgus while applying the hind part of the plaster and hence is corrected with the forefoot during gradual closure of the turn-buckle during manipulation twice a day—a single turn each time, by the mother of the affected child (Fig. 19.7). This device is applied to those feet showing resistance on manipulation. (Fig. 19.8).

Turco[56,57] advocates correction of all the components of the deformity simultaneously and not the time-honoured method of correcting the forefoot adduction first, varus next and finally the equinus. He

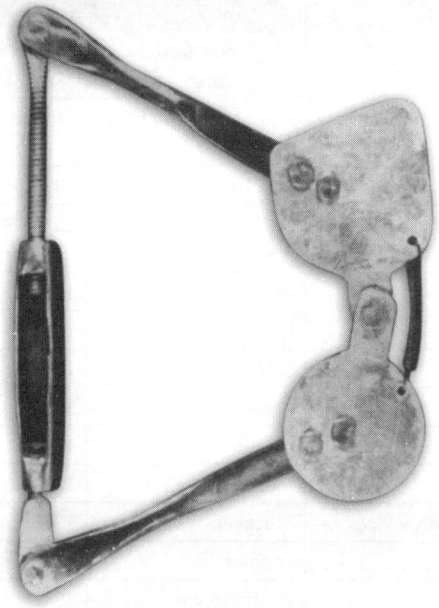

Fig. 19.5: A forefoot abduction device shown with a turnbuckle and a separate spring

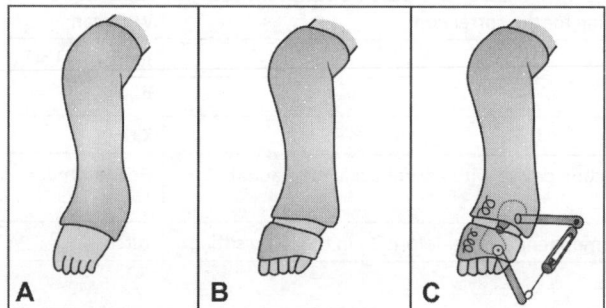

Figs 19.6A to C: The method of application of the instrument shown in three steps: (A) The hindpart of the plaster applied; (B) The forepart of the plaster applied leaving a wedge on the lateral side; (C) The instrument applied on the plantar aspect of the foot by further plastering, fixing a spring on the dorsomedial part

opines that the above deformities occur simultaneously and not as separate isolated component and hence complete correction is impossible without eliminating all the deformities at a time.

Ponseti[57] advocated manipulation of the foot followed by a long leg casting in a definite sequence. Plantar flexion of the first ray is corrected first, keeping the foot supinated inside the cast. The calcaneum is abducted, extended and everted next under the talus in a supinated foot by pressing against the head of the talus. A fully abducted foot is then dorsiflexed for the correction of equinus. Percutaneous tenotomy of tendo Achillis is often necessary. Not more than 2 to 4 casting is desirable. Denis-Browne splint is given fulltime for 3 months and at night for 2 to 4 years for maintenance of correction.

In the neonatal period, most of the club foot are corrected by the procedures mentioned. The maintenance of correction will be by application of Denis Browne splint at weekly interval three or four times. Further maintenance will be by applying hobble boots till the child learns walking, when a pair of reverse shoes is given.

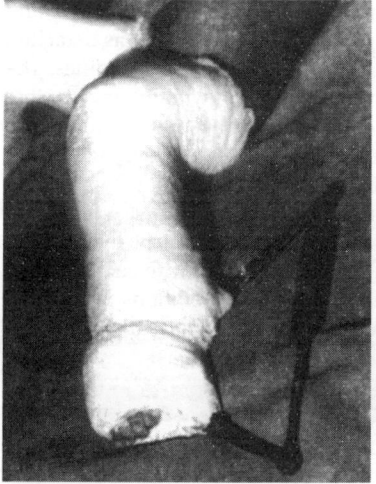 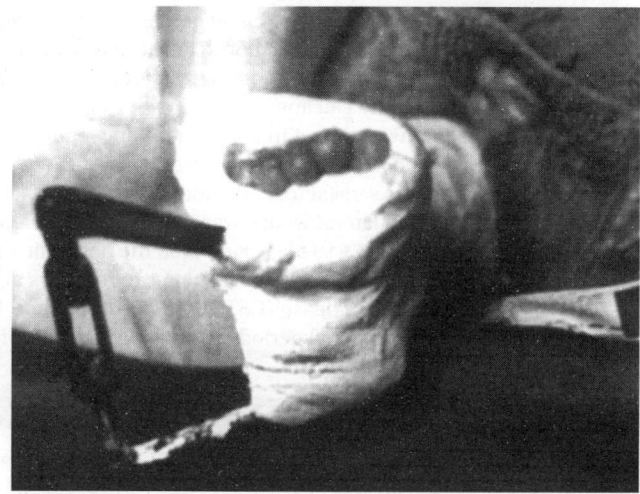

Fig. 19.7: The plastered limb with the turnbuckle

Fig. 19.8: The device applied with plaster under the sole of the deformed foot

Table 19.3: The early operative treatment of club foot	
Nature of operation	Proponent
Early operation by soft tissue release	Attenborough Apley Denham Swann, lloyd Roberts Catterall Main et al Chacko and Mathews
Operation of soft tissue release in the neonatal period	Ryoppy and Sairanen Somppi and Sulamma

Failure of conservative treatment is maintained with Denis Browne splint up to the age of 6 weeks to 3 months when operative correction is done (Table 19.3). The optimum age for surgery to produce best possible results has been talked about by many and the great proponents of early operation are Attenborough,[58] Apley,[52] Denham,[59] Swann, Lloyd Roberts and Catterall,[26] Main et al[60,61] and Chacko and Mathews[53] Operation in the neonatal period has been done by Ryoppy and Sairanen[62] from Helsinki. They primarily operated on 87 resistant club feet in 67 babies soon after birth, after the postnatal problems were looked after. The mean age of the babies at operation was 12 days—with a range of 2 to 41 days. The mean follow-up was 4.4 years with a minimum of two years with very convincing results. The early operation carried out by Somppi and Sulamma[63] was revised by Ryoppy and performed under general anaesthesia and tourniquet without using an operative microscope. Magnifying lenses were used where necessary. The talocalcaneal joint was released in 68 out of 89 feet from posterior and medial sides and partially on the lateral side cutting the tendo calcaneus in coronal plane for lengthening later on. The ligaments attached to the calcaneum on the medial side were released. The ankle joint was released posteriorly in 68 out of 89 feet and the posterior part of deltoid ligament was cut in 64 out of 89 feet. Correction of calcaneum to valgus was now possible. The forefoot correction, when not obtained, was achieved with release of plantar muscles and fascia from the calcaneum. A separate incision was made, where full correction was not achieved leaving intact skin between the medial malleolus and the calcaneum. For perfect talo-naviculocalcaneal reduction, the posterior tibial tendon was detached from the navicular and the talo-navicular and talocalcaneal joints were opened along joint lines. The foot was placed in a slightly calcaneovalgus position at the end of the operation without any forcible manipulation. The foot was placed in a moulded long leg plaster cast with the knee in flexion and the foot in calcaneovalgus position. The plaster was changed every three to six weeks. Manipulation was not done if the correction was satisfactory. The foot was immobilised in a splint from six months to walking age. A normal shoe with a lateral wedge was then used. They reported excellent result in 90% (80 out of 89 feet) and poor result in 10% (9 feet). However, the basics lie in keeping the foot in corrected position postoperativly for four months for the tarsal bones to remold stable articular surfaces with each other.[64]

The complete soft tissue release (CSTR), bony surgery and tendon transfer operations necessarily performed long after the neonatal period are not within the purview of this book and have been omitted.

REFERENCES

1. Little WJ. A Treatise on the Nature of club-foot and Analogous distortions. London; W. Jeffs, S. Highley (1839); Quoted by fripp AT and Shaw NE: Club Foot. Edinburgh and London, E & S Livingstone, 1967.p.9.
2. Hippocrates. The Genuine works of Hippocrates. Translated from the Greek by Francis Adams. Baltimore: Williams and Wikins, 1939. Quoted by Turco VJ: Clubfoot. Churchill Livingstone, 1981.p.6.
3. Wynne-Davies R. Family studies and the cause of congenital club foot. J Bone Joint Surg. 46B: 445.
4. Palmar RM. The genetics of Talipes equinovarus. J Bone Joint Sug. 1964;41B: 542.
5. Browne D. Talipes Equinovarus, Lancet. 1934;II:969-74.
6. Heuter, von Volkmann: Quoted by Fripp AT, Shaw NE. Club Foot. Edinburgh: E and S Livingstone; 1967.p.19.
7. Bassel Hagen. Quoted by Fripp AT and Shaw NE: Club Foot. Edinburgh: E & S Livingstone; 1967.p.19.
8. Bohm M. The embryologic origin of clubfoot. J Bone Joint Surg 1929;11:229.
9. Walsingham, Hughes. Quoted by Fripp AT and Shaw NE: Club Foot. Edinburgh: E & S Livingstone; 1967.
10. Irani RN, Sherman HS. The pathological anatomy of clubfoot. J Bone Joint Surg 1963;45A:45.
11. Issacs H, Handelsman JE, Badenhorst M, Pickering A. The muscles in clubfoot - a histological, histochemical and electron microscopic study. J Bone Joint Surg 1977;59B.
12. Ionasecu V, Maynard JA, Ponseti V, Zellweger H. Helvetica Paediatrica Acta 1974;29: 305 quoted by Turco VJ: Clubfoot. New York, Edinburgh, London and Melbourne: Churchill Livingstone; 1981.p.7.
13. Diaz AV. Embryological contribution to the etiopathology of Idiopathic clubfoot. J Bone Joint Surg. 1979.p.61A.
14. Scarpa A. A Memoir on the congenital clubfeet of children (translated by JW Wishart). Edinburgh, Constable, 1818.
15. Adams W. Clubfoot. Its causes, pathology and treatment. London: J & A Churchill; 1866.
16. Brockman EP. Congenital Clubfoot. Bristol: John Wright & Sons; 1930.
17. Evans D. Relapsed clubfoot: J Bone Joint Surg. 1961;43B: 722.
18. Attenborough CG. Congenital talipes equinovarus. J Bone Joint Surg. 1966;48:31-9.
19. Goldner JL. Congenital Talipes Equinovarus - Fifteen year surgical treatment. Current practice in Orthopedic Surgery CV. St. Louis: Mosby; 1962.p.4.
20. Truco VJ. Club Foot. Edinburgh: Churchill Livingstone; 1981.p.46.
21. Mckay DW. New concept of and approach to clubfoot treatment. Section I-Principles and morbid anatomy. J Pediatric Orthop 1982;2:347-56.
22. Kleiger B. The significance of tibio talar navicular complex in congenital clubfoot. Quoted by Turco VJ: Clubfoot. Edinburgh: Churchill Livingstone; 1981.p.53.
23. Simons GW. Complete subtalar release in clubfoot, Part II-comparison with less extensive procedures. J Bone Joint Surg 1985;67A:1056-65.
24. Simons GW. The complete subtalar release in clubfoot. Orthop Clin NA 1987;18(4):117.
25. Turco VJ. Clubfoot. New York: Churchill Livingstone; 1981.pp.59-83.

26. Lloyd Roberts GC, Swann M, Catterall A. Medial rotational osteotomy for severe resistant deformity in club foot. J Bone Joint Surg 1974;56B:37.
27. Swann M, Lloyd Roberts GC, Catterall A. The anatomy of the uncorrected clubfoot. J Bone Joint Surg 1969;51B:263.
28. Kite HJ. Principles involved in treatment of club foot. J Bone Joint Surg 1939;2:595.
29. Salter RB. Quoted by Mukhopadhyay B. Current Concepts in Orthopedics edited by Taneja DK. Indore: Sat Prachar Press; 1996.p.60.
30. Wynne Davies R. Family studies and the cause of congenital club foot. J Bone Joint Surg 1964.p.46B.
31. Herold J, Marcovich C. Tibial torsion in untreated congenital club foot. Acta Orthopedica Scan. 1976;47:112.
32. Pandey S, Pandey A. Clinical Orthopedic Diagnosis. New Delhi: Jaypee Brothers.
33. De Mazumder N. A New device for the correction of forefoot adduction deformity in club foot. Journal of VIMS 1978;1(1):89-90.
34. De Mazumder N, Mukherjee P. Evaluation of 73 consecutive cases of club foot treated in the club foot clinic. Journal of VIMS 1978;1(2):14-9.
35. Harold AJ, Walker CJ.
36. Srivastava, et al. Foot print analysis of club foot. Indian J Orthop 1990;24(1):13.
37. Catterall A. The club foot. London: Heinemann Medical Books Ltd; 1988.
38. McMaulay JC. History of the development and the concept of pathogenesis and treatment of club foot. Clinical Orthopedics 1972;84:25-7.
39. Hildamus Fabricius (1646) quoted by Fripp AT, Shaw NF, Club foot. Edinburgh: E & S Livingstone; 1967.p.5.
40. Arcaeus F. (1658): Ibid, 3.
41. Pare A. (1665) Quoted by Turco VJ. Club foot. New York: Churchill Livingstone; 1981.p.1.
42. Bruckner (1796) quoted by Fripp AT, Shaw NF, Club foot. Edinburgh: E & S Livingstone; 1967.p.2.
43. Forrester-Browne M. The treatment of congenital talipes equinovarus. J Bone Joint Surg 1935;661:17.
44. Lorenz (1884). Quoted by Fripp AT and Shaw NE Club foot. Edinburgh: E & S Livingstone; 1967.pp.6-20.
45. Judson: Ibid, 1892.
46. Dalton: Ibidm, 1915.
47. Thomas: Ibid, 1886
48. Browne D. Splinting for controlled movement. Clinical Orthopedics 1956;8:91.
49. Guerin (1839). Quoted by Fripp AT, Shaw NE: Club foot. Edinburgh: E & S Livingstone; 1967.p.7.
50. Whitman (1910). Ibid, 7.
51. Jones R, Lovett RW. Orthopedic Surgery: 2nd edn. London: Oxford University Press; 1929.
52. Apley AG. A System of Orthopedics and Fractures, 4th edn. London: Butterworths; 324-8.
53. Chacko V, Mathews T. Some observations in the treatment of congenital club foot. Indian J Orthop 1976;10(2):127.
54. Kite HJ. Non-operative treatment of congenital club-foot. Clinical Orthopedics and Related Research. 1972;84:29.
55. Shaw NE. Comparison of three methods of treatment of congenital clubfoot. Brit Med J 1966;I:1084-6.
56. Turco VJ. Clubfoot, New York: Churchiil Livingstone; 1981.pp.59-83.
57. Penseti IV. Common errors in the treatment of condenital club foot. International orthopaedics 1997; 21:137.
58. Attenborough CG. Early posterior soft tissue release in severe talipes equinovarus: Clin Orthop 1972;84:71-8.
59. Denham RA. Early operation for severe congenital talipes equinovarus. J Bone Joint Surg 1977;59B:116.
60. Main BJ, Crider RJ, Polk M, Lloyd Roberts GC, Swann M, Kamdar BA. The results of early operation in talipes equinovarus J Bone Joint Surg 1977;59B:337-41.
61. Main BJ, Crider RJ. An analysis of residual deformity in club foot submitted to early operation. J Bone Joint Surg 1978;60B:536.
62. Ryoppys & Sairanen H. Neonatal operative treatment of club foot. J Bone Joint Surg 1983;65B:320-5.
63. Somppi E, Sulamma M. Early operative treatment of congenital clubfoot. Acta Orthop Sand 1971;42:513-20.
64. Turco VJ. Personal communication, 1988.

Chapter 20

Arthrogryposis Multiplex Congenita

Keywords: Arthrogryposis – a group of abotu 150 syndromes of joint contractures involving all four extremities – present at birth – their types – incidence – pathology – clinical features – diagnosis – treatment.

INTRODUCTION

Arthrogryposis represents a group of about 150 syndromes, all of which have in common obvious joint contractures involving all four extremities, being present at birth. Goldberg[1] has classified them into three types. This includes arthrogryposis multiplex congenita, Larsen syndrome, and pterygia syndrome, with more or less total body involvement.

Distal arthrogryposis predominantly or exclusively involves the hands and feet. Freeman Sheldon whistling face syndrome is included, as facial involvement is combined with distal arthrogryposis.

Pterygia syndromes, in which identifiable skin webs cross the flexor aspects of the knees, elbows and other joints, are also included. Multiple pterygia and popliteal pterygium fit in this group. It is perhaps easiest to address the other syndromes if arthrogryposis multiplex congenita (amyoplasia) is first defined.

ARTHROGRYPOSIS MULTIPLEX CONGENITA

Arthrogryposis multiplex congenita is a nonprogressive clinical disorder of congenital origin, present at birth and characterized by marked stiffness and contracture of joints affecting the limbs and the trunk with improper development of muscles around them.

Although the condition was first described by Otto in 1841 as a "human wonder with curved limbs". Stern (quoted by Peter William)[2] first coined the term arthrogryposis multiplex congenita, the word arthrogryposis meaning a curved joint (Greek arthro means joint, and grypos means curved). The affected limbs lose their contours, are almost cylindrical with some joints having flexion contracture and others fixed in extension; because multiple joints are involved, Swinyard and Black[3] used the term multiple congenital contractures for this condition.

According to Sarwark, MacEwen and Scott,[4] the term should be used for a heterogenous group of disorders mimicking the condition and not for a specific diagnostic entity. On the contrary, WynneDavis, Williams and O'Conor[5] prefer to use this condition as a specific clinical entity etiologically unrelated to the arthrogryposis-like deformities of neurological disorder like myelomeningocele and myelodysplasia. The condition will be described here as two definite types as mentioned by Brown, Robson and Sharrard.[6]

Types of Arthrogryposis

Myopathic type: This type is a rare congenital non-progressive muscular dystrophy of strong hereditary predisposition of autosomal recessive type with fixed flexion contractures of limbs and gross deformities of chest and spine.[7,8,10-15]

Neuropathic type: This is due to primary neurogenic disorder of anterior horn cells with weakness or paralysis of the affected muscles, and majority of cases are sporadic in incidence with fixed extension or flexion contracture of limbs without any obvious hereditary components.[6,9]

Incidence

Arthrogryposis multiplex congenita and not "arthrogryposis-like" deformities is a rare condition and varies in incidence in different countries. The reported incidence in Helsinki was 3 per 10000 live births. In Royal Children's Hospital, Melbourne, Australia, Peter Williams detected and treated 120 cases in 20 years. A combined survey of 132 patients of arthrogryposis multiplex congenita in three different countries between 1940 and 1976 showed an occurrence of 73 from the United Kingdom, 34 from Melbourne, Australia and 25 from Delaware, USA.[2] No definite report in incidence is obtained from the orient.

Etiology

Various causative factors suggested over the years established this condition as a disease of early pregnancy associated with neurogenic, myogenic and some environmental intra-uterine factors.
1. Neurogenic cause—Joint contractures develop from muscle imbalance in early intra-uterine life, which is due to deficiency in the organization or number of anterior horn cells, roots, peripheral nerves or motor end plates.
2. Myogenic cause—Contractures are produced from non-progressive muscular dystrophy similar to that found in progressive muscular dystrophies.
3. Intra-uterine environmental factors—Hormonal, vascular, mechanical, infective and limited movements of foetus. These are mostly being incriminated as associated and not causative factors.
   Prolonged intra-uterine immobilization of joints in various stages of development of fetus in conditions like oligohydramnios, foetal malposition and in association with amniotic bands of simultaneous multiple pregnancies has been found as predisposing factor.
4. Hyperthermia—In early pregnancy, hyperthermia has been suggested as a possible teratogenic cause.[16] Infection of mother during early pregnancy by the Akabane virus causing similar contractures has been reported to occur in cattles and horses but not been confirmed in human being.[2]

Pathology

Contracted soft tissues produced deformities with varying types of adhesions in different joints. The patella is sometimes found to be fixed to the front of the femur in contracture of knee in extension. Similarly in a deformed elbow, the olecranon may be adherent with the posterior aspect of humerus.

Definite changes are observed in the muscles, nerves and in the joints.

In the muscles—Some muscles appear normal, whereas others are small or absent or replaced by fat and fibrous tissue. Sometimes, a whole muscle compartment is absent like biceps and brachialis in elbow. The more affected muscles look pale-pink. The contractures are stronger and healthier muscles overpowering their antagonists. Microscopically, the fibres are small, stain indistinctly, but retain both transverse and longitudinal striations.

In the nerves—There is fibrous infiltration of nerve bundles, peripheral nerves and anterior horn cells, which are degenerated and decreased in number; shortening is observed in the nerves contained within contracted soft tissues on the concave side of the deformity.

In the joints—Ligaments, capsules and periarticular tissues and the vessels within contracted tissues are short in length. Intra-articular tissues are contracted in an untreated case, specially in a severely affected foot the joints around the talus are poorly formed with intra-articular adhesions.[9]

Clinical Features

The clinical findings in arthrogryposis congenita have been described by different authors under various headings, and about 150 such odd syndromes may be identified.[17] Hall et al[18] found many reports on

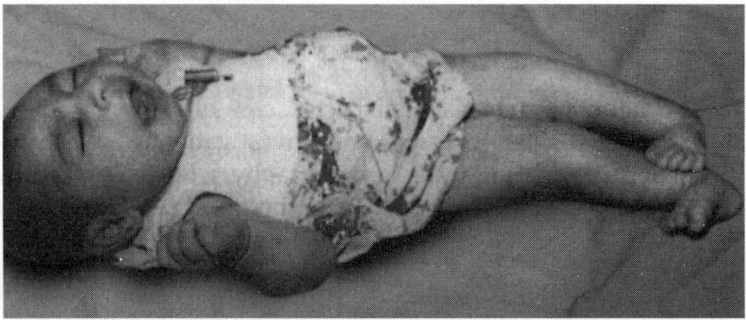

Fig. 20.1: Arthrogryposis multiplex congenita with involvement of both lower limbs—bilateral dislocation of hips, equinovarus deformity in left foot and calcaneovalgus in right foot being the features

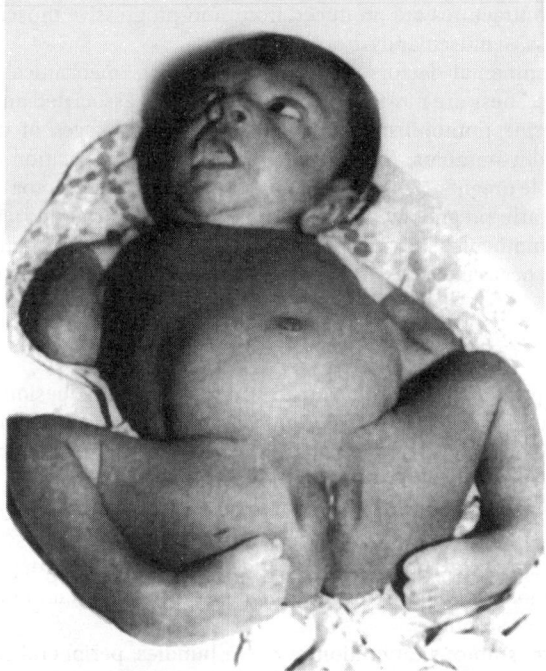

Fig. 20.2: Arthrogryposis multiplex congenita with flexion deformities in the knees, clubfeet and abduction external rotation in the hips

arthrogryposis in the European literature since the early nineteenth century. The present author treated babies with congenital arthrogryposis in a period of 22 years between 1975 and 1996. The patients were seen between birth and four years of age (Figs 20.1 and 20.2) and found to have joint contractures involving the limbs and the trunk with poor and wasted muscles around the joints. Intelligence was unimpaired in all the patients. The myopathic type is present at birth, hereditary and nonprogressive in nature, bilaterally symmetrical in involvements mostly affecting all four limbs and sometimes involving two limbs, lower extremities being more affected than the upper limbs. The affected limbs show joint contracture in flexion or extension with loss of normal contours, knobly joints, absent skin creases and deep skin dimples on or near the affected joints. Webbing is seen in the flexor aspect of the joint. Association of club foot is quite common. Congenital dislocation of hip is found on many occasions and sometimes dislocation of knee with genu recurvatum is an outcome of the condition. Scoliosis or spinabifida cystica as an associated finding is detected sometimes.

Brown, Robson and Sharard[6] found two types of arthrogryposis multiplex congenita neurological in the upper limbs, and six types in the lower limbs, each corresponding to specific cervical or lumbar involvements causing deformity from paresis or paralysis of the muscles affected, the condition is presenting at birth with the joints and the skin being same as described above. In their classical description of upper limbs involvement, they showed adduction and medial rotation of shoulder with either flexion or extension of the elbow, flexion and ulnar deviation of the wrist, and occasional weakness of intrinsics in both the types of upper limb involvement.

In the six types of lower limb affection they found flexion with or without adduction of the hip in three types with associated extension of the knee in two types and flexion of the knee in the other. Equinus with or without varus of the foot was common to all the types and in one type—a particular case with a single lower limb involvement the flexion deformity of knee was associated with equinovarus of foot. Two patients had weak intrinsic muscles of the feet. The skin sensation was normal in both upper and lower limbs. Four patients developed spinal deformity—scoliosis in three and hyperlordosis in the lumbar region in one patient.

Diagnosis

In order to come to a definite diagnosis, a suspected case of arthrogryposis should be subjected to a neurological assessment, radiographic investigation when necessary, serum enzyme study, nerve conduction studies, electromyography, where possible, and a muscle biopsy, as the arthrogrypotic syndromes mimic each other.

The two varieties of arthrogryposis—the congenital myopathic type of recessive inheritance and the neuropathic type of sporadic occurrence will have to be differentiated from other arthrogrypotic syndrome of sporadic but common occurrence-amyoplasia, manifested with multiple congenital contractures, symmetrical in nature and involving all four limbs which may have decreased girth of the muscles. Regarding the cause of this syndrome, both neuropathic and myopathic changes were observed in different muscle sites of the same patients in electromyographic studies as reported by Hall et al.[18] No anterior horn cell defect was found and histological examination of muscles revealed nonspecific changes of replacement of muscle tissue with fibrofatty scar tissue having normal muscle spindle.

Treatment

The deformities in arthrogryposis are difficult to correct as the muscles are replaced by resistible fibrous tissues. Even when a deformed limb is corrected by stretching or plastering, it is difficult to maintain the functional position as balancing muscles are often found paralysed and inadequate to hold the correction. But an attempt for correction should always be made preferably immediately after birth as the tissues stretch better at that time. A passive stretching program has been suggested followed by serial splinting. The need for corrective surgical procedures is less following this method.[16] Careful splinting and meticulous surgery are often rewarding and should be tried even in severe cases.

The principles of orthopedic treatment as suggested by Drummond, Seller and Cruess[19] and later on by William[20] are acceptable to most of the surgeons. The authors emphasized the need for establishment of muscle balance with available functioning muscles, tenotomy with capsulotomy and in more resistant cases casulotomy on contracted flexor side of the joint have been suggested, which are to be followed by holding the correction with plastering and subsequently by orthosis. The surgical procedure as suggested by them should aim at maximum correction, as wedging or corrective casts have very little role for further correction. The authors further suggested corrective osteotomies at skeletal maturity to transfer the range of the motion to a more useful arc. For the correction of clubfoot component in three feet, Joshi's external stabilization system (JESS) fixator[20] has been used by the present author between three and four years of age with good results.

Lower limb deformities—In arthrogryposis with clubfoot correction by serial plastering is done. When a functional correction is not achieved, posteromedial release may be tried usually at about the age of four to six months. An incomplete correction or recurrence of deformity will invite further correction by a drastic operation like talectomy. The results of talectomy are often good, as there is achievement of fusion between the tibia, calcaneum and navicular with age if the functional position is maintained with plaster or brace. The results of tendon transfer are not satisfactory as a good, nonfibrotic, and functioning transferable tendon is difficult to obtain. In a skeletally mature foot with a residual deformity, correction is usually obtained by tarsal or metatarsal osteotomies or by triple arthrodesis. The foot always remains small and will require a specially ordered shoe.

Failure of stretching or plaster correction of flexion contracture of knee will need surgery. Often hamstring release is inadequate, hence, a supracondylar osteotomy of femur with the base of the wedge anteriority placed will be necessary. Femoral shortening may be required to release tension in the posterior neurovascular structures. A hyperextension deformity of knee (genu recurvatum) with or without dislocation needs correction at a very early age, by quadriceps plasty and open reduction with Kirschner's wire fixation, where necessary. Stretched and attenuated anterior cruciate ligament is difficult pathology to treat with. A late case of genu recurvatum will have adaptive changes in the upper tibia, and the femoral condyles are often found square. The correction is achieved by osteotomy.

A unilateral dislocation of hip resists correction due to fibrosis, and is to be treated with open reduction because, the late result of a failed reduction is troublesome shortening of limb length with pelvic obliquity and scoliosis. Bilaterally dislocated hip should better be left alone if conservative treatment for correction fails.

Upper limb deformities—The upper limbs may be adequately functioning even in the presence of severe deformity. A failed operative treatment is often found to produce disaster. Hence, operative correction is usually not done until the age of three or four years or best deferred till skeletal maturity.[21] If need be, the shoulder deformity of adduction, and internal rotation is corrected by upper humeral rotational osteotomy. To help the patient feeding on his or her own, the elbow flexion needs reinforcement by triceps transfer to radial neck or by a Steindler proximal transportation of flexors of forearms.[22] Often the elbow may need fusion after skeletal maturity. A palmar flexion deformity of wrist and hand can be corrected by a Riordan-like procedure of centralization of radial clubhand and at skeletal maturity by wrist fusion, when spontaneous carpal fusion is commonly found. In the fingers, a combination of stiff metacarpophalangeal or interphalangeal joints with absent or weak long flexors and extensors is often found. The results of surgery like sublimis transfer or dorsal release of interphalangeal joints or metacarpal osteotomies are poor in these conditions. However, a hypoplastic thumb clasped into the palm can be corrected by release of the web, a skin supplementation and a tendon transfer to the dorsum to replace the absent extensors and abductors.

Scoliosis—Ten to thirty per cent patients with arthrogryposis present with scoliosis.[23] As mentioned before, the deformity is associated with pelvic obliquity due to unilateral dislocation of hip. Correction with plasters and braces should be tried at an early age.

The results of treatment in arthrogryposis are not at all rewarding. The object of treatment is defeated if a patient cannot be made to stand or walk and do his or her usual work. The results of treatment of 75 patients with lower extremity arthrogryposis[24] reveals a not too gloomy picture, where 50 per cent walked independently following operations, 25 per cent walked with braces and 25 per cent were bedridden or led wheel-chair life.

OTHER FORMS OF ARTHROGRYPOSIS

Larsen syndrome, distal arthrogryposis, Freeman Sheldon syndrome, and the pterygia syndromes have joint contractures, dislocations, and deformities that are similar to classic arthrogryposis multiplex congenita, but they also have several distinctive features.

Characteristic features of Larsen syndrome are multiple congenital dislocations of large joints, a characteristic flat face, and ligamentous laxity.[25] It is a hereditary disorder. Common joints dislocated are the knees, the hips and the elbows. The dislocation is usually bilateral, caused by ligamentous laxity. Patient may have bilateral clubfeet. The primary treatment is to reduce the joint with or without operation. If an infant is brought early, close manipulation of the dislocated joint may succeed. All other deformities are treated with osteotomies, tendon transfers or soft tissue release. Differential diagnosis of multiple congenital dislocations are: (i) Larsen syndrome, (ii) Marfan's syndrome, (iii) Congenital laxity of joints, and (iv) Achler's Dunlop syndrome.

Distal Arthrogryposis

Children with distal arthrogryposis have characteristic fixed hand contractures and foot deformities, but the major large joints of the arms and legs are spared.[26,27,4] The deformities of the hand are ulnar deviation of finger, flexion deformities of the finger joints and adducted thumb; the foot may have Talipesequino varus or vertical talus.

Freeman-Sheldon Syndrome

"Freeman-Sheldon syndrome" is often combined with distal arthrogryposis. It is recognized by its most characteristic feature, a "whistling face". Scoliosis is common.

Pterygia Syndrome

Pterygium comes from a Greek word meaning little wing. A pterygium is a web. There are clinically important pterygia syndromes: (i) multiple pterygia syndrome, and (ii) popliteal pterygia syndrome.[28] Popliteal web is common. Surgery is rarely needed for the upper extremities. Early surgery for the web, especially in popliteal region is recommended. There is high recurrence rate despite previous surgery. Femoral shortening and extension osteotomy were considered previously.

OTHER ORTHOPEDICALLY IMPORTANT SYNDROMES WITH JOINT CONTRACTURES, DISLOCATIONS AND DEFORMITIES PRESENT AT BIRTH

Fetal Alcohol Syndrome

Infant born of alcoholic mothers, who drink throughout pregnancy may have malformations. Alcohol is considered as a teratogen. A cardinal clinical feature is disturbed growth. Growth retardation starts in the intrauterine period continues in childhood despite good nutrition. The second important feature is disturbed central nervous system development. The child may present as a case of cerebral palsy, hypotonia or spasticity. Orthopedic problems are stiffness of the hand, a club-foot, dysplasia of the hip and fusion of the cervical vertebrae.

Noonan Syndrome

In Noonan syndrome, the patient has similar clinical features. However, the chromosomes are normal. The syndrome affects both boys and girls. The incidence is 1 in 1000, and it is an autosomal dominant disorder.[29]

Down Syndrome

Down syndrome is the most common and perhaps the most readily recognizable malformation in humans. Complete trisomy 21 accounts for 95 per cent of the cases, with 2 per cent mosaics and 3 per cent translocations. The overall risk is 1 per 660 live births, and the incidence is closely related to maternal age. If the mother is younger than 30 years of age, the risk is 1 in 5000 live births, and if the mother is older than 35 years of age, the incidence rises to 1 in 250.[30]

The classic features are characteristic facies, hand anomalies, congenital heart disease, and some aspects of the mental retardation results from the duplication of a single band, 21q 22.2-22.3.[17] About one-half of the patients with Down syndrome have scoliosis, with an idiopathic pattern in 99 per cent.[31] The pelvis of an infant with Down syndrome has a diagnostic roetgenographic appearance characterized by flat acetabula and flared iliac wings. There may be deformities in the joints. The patient has a short stature.

REFERENCES

1. Goldberg MJ. Syndromes of Orthopedic Importance. In Morissy RT and Weinstein ST (Eds): Pediatric Orthopedics by Lovell and Winter's (4th edn) 1996;1:262.
2. William P. The management of arthrogryposis. Orthop Clin North Am 1978;9:67-8.
3. Swinyeard CA, Black EE. The Etiology of Arthrogryposis (Multiple congenital contracture). Clin Orthop 1985;194:74.
4. Sarwark F, MacEwen Dean G, Scott I. Amyoplasia (a common form of arthrogryposis) - current concepts review. JBJS, 1990;72(A): 465-9.
5. Wynne-Davis Ruth, Williams, O'conor JCB. The 1960s epidemic of arthrogryposis multiplex congenital - a survey from the United Kingdom, Australia and the United Sates of America. JBJS 1981;64B: 76-82.
6. Brown LM, Robson MJ, Sharrard WJM. The pathophysiology of arthrogryposis multiplex congenita neurologica. JBJS 1980;62B: 261-96.
7. Banker BQ, Victor M, Adams RD. Arthrogryposis due to congenital muscular dystrophy. Brain, 1958;80: 319-34.
8. Drachman DB, Banker BQ (1961). Quoted by Brown et al. JBJS 1980;62B: 291-6.
9. Krugliak L, Gadoth N, Behar AJ. Neuropathic form of arthrogryposis multiplex congenita. JBJS 1980;62B: 291-6.
10. Lebenthal F, Schochet SB, Adam A, et al. Arthrogryposis multiplex congenita - 23 cases in an Arab kindred. Pediatrics 1970;46:891-99.
11. Mead NG, Lithgow NC, Sweency HJ. Arthrogryposis multiplex congenita. JBJS 1958;40a:1285-1309.
12. Greenfield JG, Common T, Shy GM. The prognostic value of muscle in the floppy infant Brain, 1958;81: 461-84.
13. Pearson CM, Fowler WG (Jr.). Hereditary non-progressive muscular dystrophy inducing arthrogryposis syndrome. Brain, 1963;86:75-88.
14. Stoeber E (1938). Quoted by Brown et al. JBJS 1980;62B: 291-6.
15. Ullrich O (1938). Quoted by Brown et al. JBJS 1980;62B: 291-6.
16. Palmer PM, MacEwan GD, Bowen JR, et al. Passive motion for infants with arthrogryposis. Clin Orthop 1994;54: 1985.
17. Brock DJH. Molecular Genetics for the Clinician. Cambridge: Cambridge University Press; 1993.

18. Hall JG, Reed SD, Driscoll EP. Part I, Amyoplasia - a common sporadic condition with congenital contracture. Quoted by Sarward JF, MacEwen DG, Scott CI. JBJS 1990;62A: 465-9.
19. Drummond DS, Seller TN, Cruess RL. The management of arthrogryposis multiplex congenita. In American Academy of Orthopedic Surgeons: Instructional course lectures 23. St. Louis: CV Mosby; 1974. 73 (quoted from Cambell's Operative Orthopedics, edn by AH Crenshaw; 7th edn, St. Louis: CV Mosby; 4:3038.
20. Joshi BB, Laud NS, Warrier SS, Kanaji BG, Joshi AP, Debake H. Treatment of CTEV by Joshi's external stabilization system (JESS). In G.S. Kulkarni (Ed) Text Book of Orthopedics and Trauma, Vol 2. New Delhi: Jaypee Brothers Medical Publishers (P) Ltd 1999;21:1475-984.
21. Shapiro Bresnan. Operative management of childhood neuromuscular disease, current concepts review part II - peripheral neuropathies. Firedreich's ataxia and arthrogryposis multiplex congenita. JBJS 1982;64A: 951-3.
22. Tachdjian MO. Pediatric Orthopedics. Philadelphia: WB Saunders; 1978.
23. Drummond DS, Mackenzie DA. Scoliosis in arthrogryposis multiplex congenita. Spine 1978;3:146-51.
24. Gibson DA, Urs NDK. Arthrogryposis multiplex congenita. JBJS 1970;52B:483-93.
25. Larsen LJ, Schottsstaedt ER, Bost FC. Multiple congenital dislocation associated with characteristic facial abnormality. J Pediatr 1950;37:574.
26. Dhaliwal AS, Myers TL. Digitotalar dysmorphism. Orthop Rev 1985;14:90.
27. Salis JG, Beighton P. Dominantly inherited digitotalar dysmorphism. JBJS 1972;54B:509.
28. Hall JG, Reed SD, Resenbaum KN, et al. Limb pterygium syndromes—a review and report of 11 patients. Am J Med Genet 1982;12:377.
29. Sharlond M, Morgan M, Smith G, et al. Genetic counselling in Noonan syndrome, Am J Med Genet 1993;45: 437.
30. Gath A. A parental reactions to loss and disappointment - the diagnosis of Down's syndrome. Dev and Child Neurol 1985;27:932.
31. Diamond LS, Lynne D, Sigman B. Orthopedic disorders in patients with Down's syndromes. Orthop Clin N Am 1981;12:57.

Chapter 21

Congenital Subluxations and Dislocations Around the Knee

Keywords: Congenital subluxations and dislocations around the knee in a neonate—isolated or part of a syndrome—three grades—treatment is conservative or operative to improve flexion of the knee.

CONGENITAL SUBLUXATIONS AND DISLOCATIONS AROUND THE KNEE

Congenital genu recurvatum or congenital dislocation or subluxation of the knee in a neonate is variation of a congenitally hyperextended knee. The baby is often delivered vaginally as a case of breech presentation or sometimes the delivery is through caesarean section. Often multiple dislocations of different joints are associated as a part of a syndrome like Larsen or Down or Ehlers-Danlos. The deformity may be part of dislocations of hip and knee due to arthrogryposis multiplex congenita and the feet may also be deformed into talipes equino varus or convex pes valgus or calcaneus (Fig. 21.1). Other anomalies like imperforate anus, cryptorchidism, spina bifida, hydrocephalus, cleft palate, facial paralysis are often associated. In a clear case of subluxation or dislocation of the knee routine anteroposterior and lateral radiograph clinch the diagnosis.

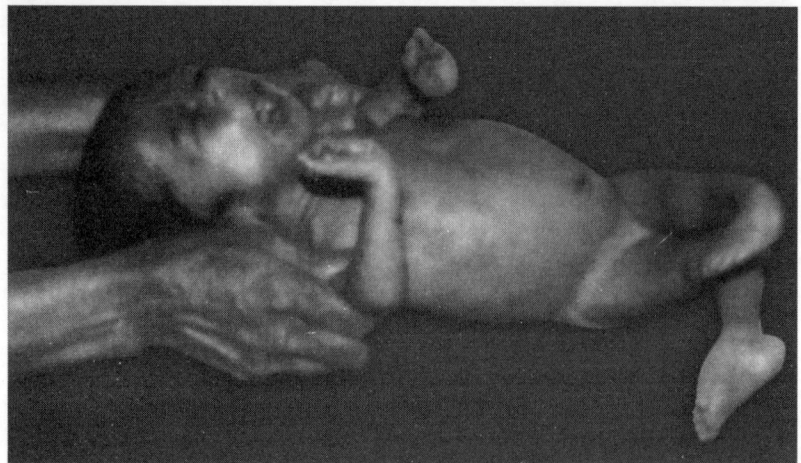

Fig. 21.1: The congenital dislocation of knee of right side as a part of arthrogryposis multiplex congenita and the left foot showing club foot deformity

Congenital Subluxations and Dislocations Around the Knee

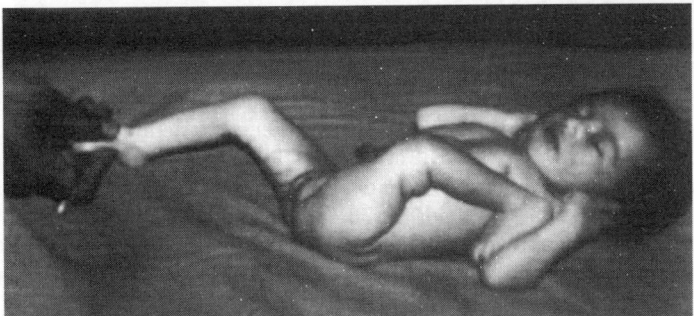

Fig. 21.2: Congenital subluxation of the left knee of grade II

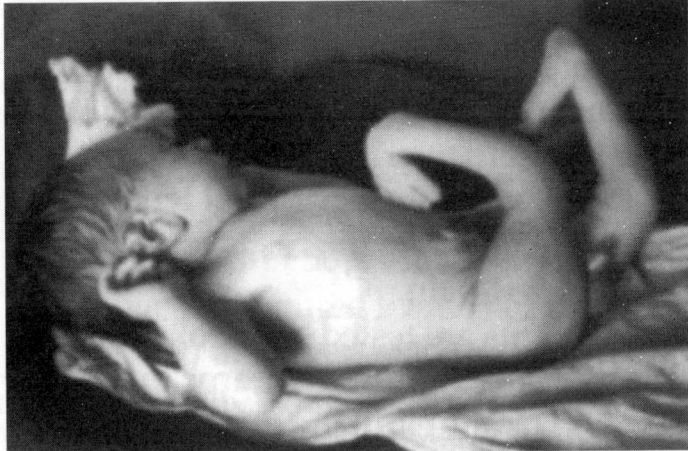

Fig. 21.3A: Bilateral congenital subluxation of the knees with dislocation in the right hip

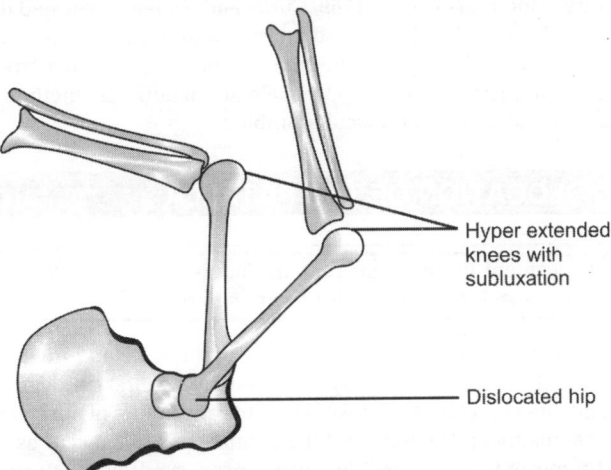

Fig. 21.3B: Bilateral congenital subluxation of the knees and dislocation in the right hip shown diagrammatically

But, it is often difficult in a neonate to differentiate the deformity into its real grade. Leveuf and Pais's classification often help us to divide the deformity into grade I, where the knee can be passively flexed up to 45 to 60° beyond neutral but on release of pressure bounces back to 10 to 20° of hyperextension. There is practically no anterior displacement of tibia. In grade II, the knee is positioned at 20 to 40° of hyperextension and on passive flexion the knee is straightened to neutral position only. The anterior subluxation of tibia is moderate here (Figs 21.2 and 21.3A and B). In grade III, there is no contact between the tibia and femur in the formation of knee joint developing into total anterior dislocation.

It is not very easy to differentiate the deformity into different grades but the only noninvasive method for distinguishing is ultrasonography. A computed sonographic method clearly depicts the cartilaginous relationship of upper tibia and lower femur. Other methods like arthrography and magnetic resonance imaging are tried when the baby grows older.

Pathology

The crux of the pathology is subluxation or dislocation or simple hyperextension. Whether the associated deformities of the intrinsic and extrinsic structures of the knee are primary or secondary have been the point of research for many years. Degeneration of quadriceps muscles in the utero has been suggested by Middleton.[1] However, the condition in established case shows contracture of quadriceps, shortened patellar tendon with varying degrees of genu valgus associated with contracture of lateral intermuscular septum and iliotibial band. The suprapatellar pouch is often obliterated with hypoplastic patella. The hamstrings specially medial ones are displaced anteriorly acting like extensors. The cruciates are often absent and the collaterals are anteriorly displaced.

Treatment

Treatment should be started early in the neonatal period in order to improve flexion of the knee, which is easily achieved in grade I. Repeated manipulation and anterior plaster slab application is the method of choice. Maintenance of correction is by dynamic splinting by application of Pavlik harness or by repeated manipulation. The associated dislocation of hip is also corrected by this method of harness treatment. Failed cases will need open reduction. In grade II and III, correction is difficult to achieve by conservative means. Open reduction with elongation of contracted anterior structures of knee along with anterior capsulotomy has been recommended by authors like Niebauer and King[2] in the seventh decade of the last century. Nine years later in 1969, Curtis and Fisher[3] advocated division of quadriceps above the level of the patella by inverted V-shaped incision and release of the muscles obtained in the process. All these operations are done in older children. The other method of correction following failed method of manipulation and plastering is to apply skeletal traction. The method, however, is not free from complications like skin sloughing and vascular problem.

CONGENITAL DISLOCATION OF THE PATELLA

Keywords: Lateral displacement of the quadriceps mechanism detected clinically and by USG and MRI–treated by surgery, as closed reduction ends up with failure.

A newborn infant presenting with fixed flexion deformity of the knee and excessive lateral rotation of the tibia must have the patella displaced laterally on the lateral femoral condyle. The condition may be unilateral or bilateral and often familial. The cause is intrauterine failure of normal medial rotation of the myotome containing the quadriceps femoris and the patella. This may occur as an isolated deformity or part of multiple chromosomal abnormalities, like Larsen syndrome or arthrogryposis multiplex congenita or Down syndrome.

The nonappearance of patellar ossific center before 3 to 4 years of age makes the diagnosis of the condition difficult in the neonatal period. Ultrasonography may show the quadriceps mechanism displaced laterally from the normal anterior position on underdeveloped lateral femoral condyle. MRI helps when the child grows to six months of age.

Closed reduction is bound to end up with failure as the internal contracted structures and the lateral position of quadriceps need correction for realigning the patella into proper position. The operation by Gabazzi-Dewar[4] is done between 6 and 12 months of age of the baby, where after proper alignment of patella, semitendinous tendon is transferred to the patella after medial capsular plication with imbrication along with hemisection of the patellar tendon and transfer of the lateral half medially. In another operation done by Stanisavljevic et al[5] semitendinous tendon is not transferred, instead, after the preliminary part of realignment of the patella, a medial capsular flap is drawn anteriorly and laterally over the patella and sutured to the lateral edge of the bone. They recommend this operation to be done as soon as diagnosis is made.

REFERENCES

1. Middleton DS. The pathology of congenital genn recurvatum, Br J Surg 1935;22: 696,
2. Niebauer JJ, King DE. Congenital dislocation of the knee, J Bone Joint Surg 1960;42-A: 207.
3. Curtis BH, Fisher RL. Congenital hyperextension with anterior subluxation of the knee: surgical treatment and long-term observations. J Bone Joint Surg 1969;51-A: 255.
4. Gabazzi-Dewar. Clinical Pediatric Orthopedics—the art of diagnosis and principles of management by Mihran O Tachji, 1997, 91.
5. Stanisavljevic S, Zemenick G, Miller D. Congenital irreducible permanent lateral dislocation of the patella, Clin Orth 1976;116: 190.

Chapter 22

Developmental Dysplasia of the Hip

> **Keywords:** Dysplasia of the hip is development—absence of dislocation at birth in many - mechanical, physiological, genetic and postnatal environmental etiological factors—early diagnosis is important but difficult—straight X-Ray and USG are helpful—treatment is conservative and operative.

DEVELOPMENTAL DYSPLASIA OF THE HIP

The term developmental dysplasia of the hip (DDH) is preferred to congenital dislocation of hip (CDH) as in many children the hip is undislocated at birth but later on develops dislocation or subluxation. This is a progressive deformation of the hip, where the acetabulum, the capsule and the proximal femur with its muscles and ligaments are at fault. The femoral head displacement may occur in utero (foetal or prenatal), at birth (perinatal) or after birth (postnatal). The importance of early neonatal diagnosis of DDH has been stressed by Roser, LeDamaney and Putti.[1]

Incidence

The incidence of congenital hip instability varies from country to country. Where the incidence is low as 4.16 per 1000 live births in New Zealand, it is high in England 17 per 1000 live births.[2] However, certain factors are considered while discussing incidence, which are as follows:
1. DDH is more common in some families.
2. Relatives of children with hip dysplasia have had lax ligaments and slightly shallow acetabulum.
3. *Ethnic factor:* Incidence is 25-50 per thousand in Lapps and North American Indians, but low incidence in Chinese and Black Africans.

    A prospective study conducted by Danielsson[3] in Sweden on 24101 newborn infants for neonatal instability of the hip showed 63 per cent of parents were of Swedish extraction and 24 per cent of parents were born in a foreign country. They were further subdivided into ethnic and geographical subgroups. There was a marginal increase in incidence of dislocatable i.e., unstable hips (7.6%) among Swedish than in other geographical groups (5.8%).
4. *Environment:* High incidence in certain ethnic groups due to unnatural excessive early hip extension by infant swaddling and by use of cradle boards.
5. *Breech presentation:* A difficult intrauterine position, gradually deform the acetabular cartilaginous rim or labrum leading to dislocation or a dislocatable or subluxable hip.

Developmental Dysplasia of the Hip

Etiology

The etiology is multifactorial:
1. Mechanical
2. Physiological
3. Genetic and
4. Postnatal environmental

Mechanical

(a) Pelvis of the foetus trapped in the maternal pelvis; (b) tight maternal abdominal and uterine musculature preventing foetal movement; (c) breech presentation in about 30 to 50% cases help as mechanical factors in the causation of DDH.

Physiological

There are some physiological factors as the following which help in the causation of DDH. The suggestive factors are: (a) maternal oestrogens and other hormones causing pelvic relaxation prior to delivery; (b) increased urinary excretion of oestrone and oestradiol in the first week after birth in babies with DDH; (c) oestrogens block the synthesis of newly synthesized collagen; (d) familial incidence of about 20 percent may be due to inborn error of estrogen metabolism.

Genetic

(a) Acetabular dysplasia of polygenic inheritance; (b) joint laxity of dominant inheritance; (c) geographical incidence and (d) 20 per cent familial incidence of DDH.

Post-natal Environmental Factors

(a) Customary wrapping or swaddling in the first few months goes against the neonatal physiological position of the hip of flexion and abduction—DDH is ten times greater among them; (b) holding the newborn by feet at delivery forces, the hip in extension causing dislocation.

Pathology

A. The pathological changes in the components of the hip in congenital subluxation are:
   i. The acetabular fossa is shallow and small, looks oval or triangular in shape and the roof or superior portion is oblique, even vertical, offering no resistance to the upward migration of the head by the muscle pull or weight bearing—the acetabular dysplasia.
   ii. The superior acetabular pole is notched and irregular due to constant friction and here the labrum and the reflected tendon of the rectus femoris are pushed against the ilium and become attenuated.
   iii. The femoral head is enlarged in comparison to the small size of the acetabular fossa, and hence is difficult to be adapted to the inadequate socket.
   iv. The capsule is thickened and stretched enlarging the joint cavity to accommodate the movement of its contents.
   v. The ligamentum teres may be elongated, hypertrophied, degenerated, attenuated or absent.
   vi. The anteversion of the femoral neck is often increased.
   vii. The inferior and central portion of the acetabular fossa may be filled with fibrofatty tissue.

B. The pathological changes in the congenital dislocation of the hip:
   i. The femoral head is completely displaced out of the acetabulum and comes to rest against the lateral wall of the ilium—which, most commonly, according to Howarth,[4] lies adjacent to the anterior inferior iliac spine and secondarily comes to lie in the posterior area near the sciatic foramen.
   ii. The pressure of the head against the ilium causes the former to be flattened posteriorly and the femoral neck becomes more anteverted.
   iii. The capsule is hypertrophied and stretched helping in perpetuation of dislocation.
   iv. The upwardly pulled up capsule drags the transverse ligament up and both the capsule and the ligament become adherent to the floor of the fossa and obstruct relocation of the head. The capsule is also adherent to the ilium above.
   v. A false acetabulum or a secondary socket is formed later on at the supra-acetabular area due to pressure of the head against the ilium causing the capsule and the periosteum to differentiate into a fibrocartilaginous tissue lining a depression or socket in the bone.
   vi. Factors obstructing relocation of the head into the acetabular fossa (Fig. 22.1):
      a. Hypertrophied ligamentum teres
      b. Thick and everted glenoidal labrum
      c. Iliopsoas tendon crossing under the capsule causing an hourglass constriction
      d. Reflected head of rectus femoris tendon occasionally causing obstruction
      e. The muscles and fasciae proximal to the hip and inserting below the hip are all contracted causing difficulty in reduction of dislocation.

LeDamaney[5] suggested that the reciprocal relationship between the degree of acetabular anteversion and that of femoral anteversion when breaks down and the combination of two readings was more than 60°, instability of the hip would result. Normally, the acetabular anteversion is -2° to 16° (mean 7°) and femoral anteversion is 15° to 47°[6] Mckibbin[7] confirmed LeDamaney's observations that the acetabulum, which was shallow at birth was most unstable and susceptible to extrinsic factors helping in development of dislocation. The shallowness of the hip, they claimed, was due to increased mobility required at that time.

Difficulty in the Early Diagnosis of Developmental Dysplasia of the Hip

Diagnosis

Each and every baby kept in the hospital nursery after birth should be searched for the risk factors of DDH. The baby should undergo a screening program for the hip in order to detect early the presence

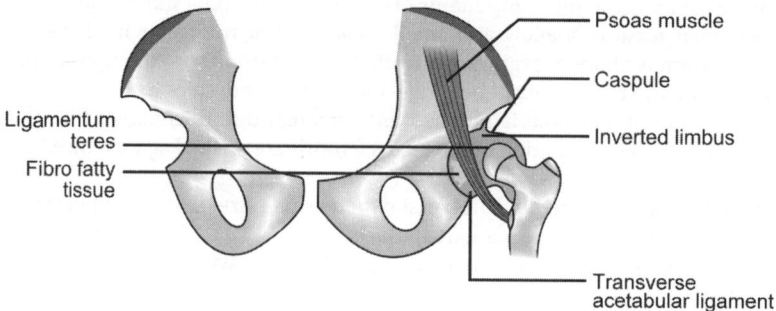

Fig. 22.1: Structural impediments to the relocation of the head of the femur into the acetabulum

of dysplasia. The reason being, DDH diagnosed late is a difficult condition to treat with. Furthermore, early diagnosis within three months of birth by clinical methods needs some specific conditions and experienced hands followed by ultrasonography by an expert sonologist for the corroboration of the presence of dysplasia. In spite of best efforts one may miss the diagnosis of DDH due to tightness of muscles around the hip or from failure of relaxation of muscles of the hip at the time of examination—a condition known as "Ilfeld phenomenon".[8]

Risk Factors

The conditions which raise suspicion or the risk factors are breech presentation, female or first born baby, family history of DDH, presence of deformities in the foot like metatarsus varus or club foot or calcaneovalgus, or some deformities in the neck like torticollis, some congenital anomalies in the heart or kidney or presence of any syndrome. A baby with suspicion of DDH should be doubly checked clinically, preferably by two experienced doctors in order to avoid a missed diagnosis.

Problems in the Diagnosis in the Newborn

The diagnosis is difficult in the newborn because of a crying baby, a tense or a hungry baby, a cursory examination by a busy doctor, examination by inexperienced hands, too firm a grip on the thigh during the examination and for improper understanding of the Ortolani and Barlow tests.

Physical Examination of the Baby

The examination should be done on a quiet or sleeping baby in a placid atmosphere and not on a hungry baby. Besides observing asymmetrical skin folds on the groin, on the medial aspect of the thigh or in the popliteal region of the suspected side and apparent shortening of the femur (Galeazzi sign), other clinical methods are those of Ortolani[9] and Barlow.[10]

The Ortolani manoeuvre is to produce reduction of dislocation by gently manipulating the head of the femur into the acetabulum crossing its rim by abducting the thigh with a soft hand hearing a clunk of entry during the process. This is not a click, which is a short, high-pitched sound caused by ligamentous or myofascial `pop' from the iliotibial band or gluteal tendons or by a vacuum phenomenon in the hip. A click is not a clinical sign of developmental dysplasia of the hip.[11]

The Barlow procedure is manoeuvering the head of the femur into dislocation by adducting the thigh. Sometimes clunk is not heard but ridge sign of the head of the femur moving over the labrum can be felt. Often relaxation after five or ten minutes produce a positive diagnosis, which was negative on first examination.

The hip after physical examination may be detected as normal or subluxatable with capsular laxity or dislocatable, i.e. Barlow positive, or dislocated. The dislocated hip may be reducible or Ortolani positive or non-reducible, i.e. teratologic. A teratologic hip is associated with severe malformations like myelomeningocele, arthrogryposis multiplex congenita, lumbosacral agenesis and chromosomal abnormalities. A nonteratologic dislocated hip sometimes may not show demonstrable movement of the head of the femur. The physical finding detected in such an irreducible hip is limitation of abduction of the flexed hip. The stiffness encountered may be the early sign of detection of dislocation and therefore, the diagnosis of such a dislocation is easily missed.

Straight X-ray

In a straight X-ray of the pelvis having both hips with the lower limbs parallel to each other and in identical position, the diagnosis of DDH is easy when the hip stands away (Fig. 22.2). The difficulty lies with those babies within six months of age, when the capital epiphysis is not ossified and the hip is subluxated and

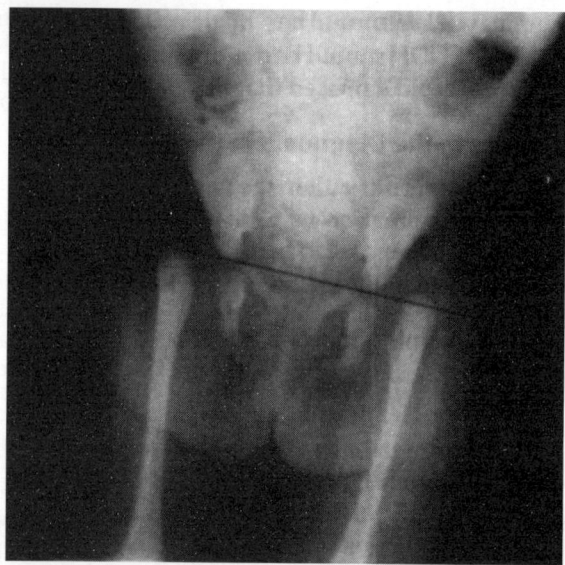

Fig. 22.2: The straight X-ray of the pelvis including the hips having both the lower limbs parallel and in identical position is diagnostic of bilateral DDH as the hips stand away

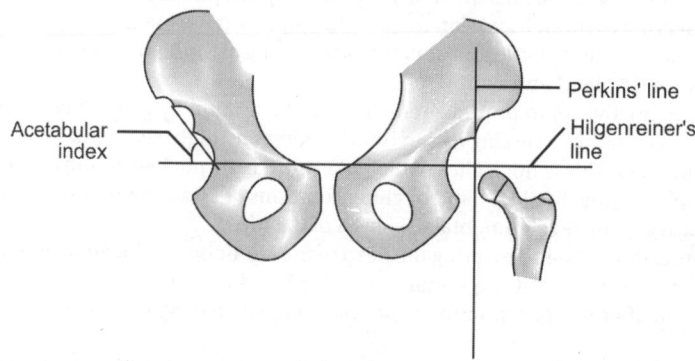

Fig. 22.3: Quadrants formed by the Perkins' and Hilgenreiner's lines expressed here by line diagram denoting subluxation when the upper femoral metaphysis is outside the lower inner quadrant

not dislocated. The drawing of Hilgenriner's and Perkin's lines on the straight X-ray shows the presence of medial beak of upper femoral metaphysis outside the lower inner quadrant in a subluxated hip (Fig. 22.3). The disruption of Shenton's line, diminution of CE angle and widening and delayed ossification of the teardrop also help in the diagnosis. Acetabular index of more than 40° is indicative of DDH (Fig. 22.4). Incidentally a cup-shaped notch immediately above the acetabulum in the lateral iliac wall appears along with steep inclination of acetabular roof in a case of DDH.[12] Because of improper degree (not 45°) of abduction and internal rotation maintained during X-ray in vonRosen's view, this is not followed by many surgeons.

Developmental Dysplasia of the Hip

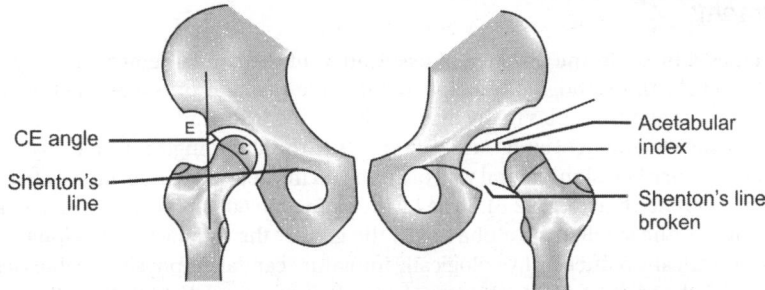

Fig. 22.4: CE angle, acetabular index and Shenton's line (broken on left side)

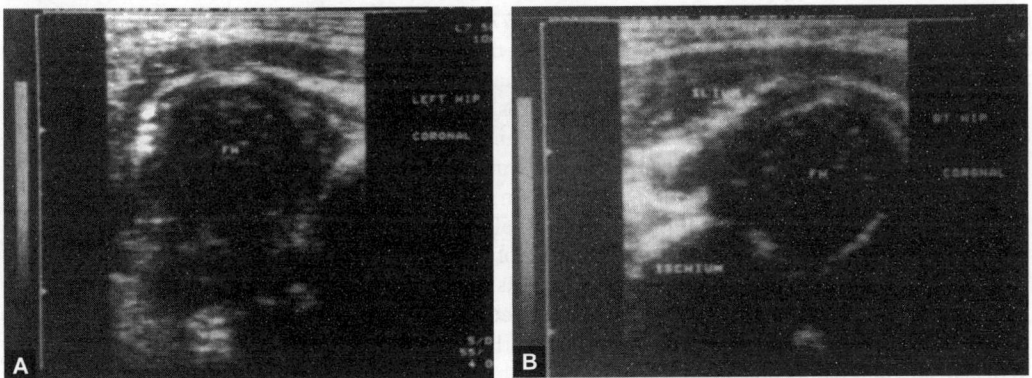

Figs 22.5A and B: Position of non-ossified capital epiphysis shown in ultrasonography

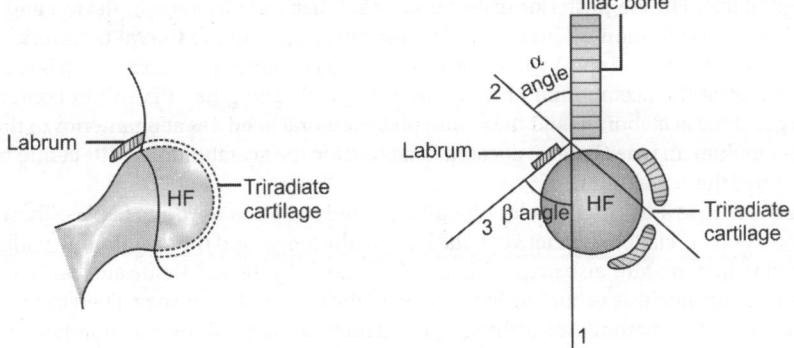

Fig. 22.6: Graf's method of quantitative ultrasonographic measurement of alpha and beta angles
  1 – Reference line, parallel to the lateral wall of ilium
  2 – Tangent line – from bony roof to the triradiate cartilage
  3 – Line from lateral bony edge of acetabulum to the labrum
  HF – Head of the femur

Ultrasonography

Diagnosis becomes difficult in the absence of ossification of the capital femoral epiphysis in the first few months after birth. Ultrasonography helps to show the position of nonossified capital epiphysis (Figs. 22.5A and B). The abnormalities in the hips are diagnosed with gradation of dysplasia according to Graf's quantitative measurement of alpha and beta angles.[13] The alpha angle is formed by a bony roof line with the vertical reference line along lateral wall of ilium and the beta angle is formed by the cartilaginous roof line with the reference line (Fig. 22.6). Type I with more than 60° alpha angle and less than 77° beta angle is a normal hip. The smaller the alpha angle, the greater the dysplasia. The alpha angle of 50° to 60° denotes, concentrically reduced physiologically immature capital epiphysis in babies less than three months old (Type IIa) and delayed ossification of capital epiphysis in babies more than three months of age (Type IIb).[14] An alpha angle between 43° and 49° indicates concentric position of cartilaginous capital epiphysis with grossly deficient acetabulum (Type IIc). Up to these values of alpha angles the beta angle remains less than 77° in first three subtypes of type II. When the value of alpha angle is between 43° and 49° but the beta angle is more than 77° it is a subluxation (Type IId). In a low dislocation, the alpha angle is less than 43° and the beta angle is more than 77° and in a high dislocation the beta angle remains as before but the alpha angle is diminutive indicating thereby gross dysplasia of bony acetabulum. These measurements are done on ultrasonography in coronal plane as nonstress static technique.[13]

Sometimes difficulty arises in arriving at a diagnosis by static methods, when dynamic stress method of ultrasonographic study[15] is done in transverse plane with the hip in neutral and in coronal plane to note the relationship of the femoral head with the acetabulum while performing Barlow or Ortolani maneuver. Up to 6 mm motion in left hip and 4 mm in right hip is normal.

The relationship between the nonossified head of the femur with the acetabulum and the pubis is assessed by Suzuki's technique of anterior imaging of both hips with ultrasonography.[16,17] A baby with DDH treated in Pavlik harness is investigated by this method to know the maintenance of reduction. The examination is done at first with the hips extended and then flexed and abducted. In extension, the femoral head is not dislocated posteriorly but anteriorly; posterior subluxation or dislocation is observed in flexion and abduction. Suzuki observed relationship of nonossified capital femoral epiphysis with the pelvis by drawing a line along the anterior surface of the pubic bones in coronal plane and with a line through the centre of the pubic bones and again with another line through the lateral margin of the pubic bone perpendicular to the anterior line and in sagittal planes. The nonossified femoral head lies posterior to the anterior line in the coronal plane keeping a very narrow space and having no space between it and the lateral sagittal line. For the posterior dislocation or subluxation observed in flexion and abduction Suzuki described a classification of three types by ultrasonography in the frontal transverse plane with the hips flexed and abducted—Type A where the posteriorly and laterally subluxated hip is still in contact with the inner wall of the acetabulum and in type B the dislocating head is still in contact with the posterior margin of the acetabulum and the centre of the femoral head lies at or anterior to the posterior edge of the acetabulum. In type C, the dislocated head outside the acetabulum has its centre posterior to the posterior rim of the acetabulum.

CT scan and MRI are advocated in older infants to avoid radiation to young babies. These, however, give good impression or relationship between the head of the femur and the acetabulum within a plaster cast after closed reduction. MRI also helps to know about not only the soft tissue and cartilaginous head but also any ischaemic necrosis occurring in the head of the femur. The cause of a persistent dislocation may be detected by the methods of arthrography, which helps to show the fibrofatty tissue filled acetabulum and the inverted limbus.

After three months of age of the baby, the diagnosis is not that difficult because of progressive contracture of the adductors, laterally rotated affected hip with positive galeazzi and telescoping sign, though Ortolani test may be negative.

Developmental Dysplasia of the Hip

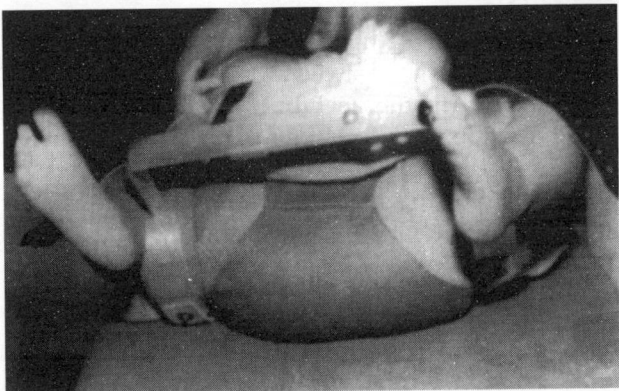

Fig. 22.7: Craig splint

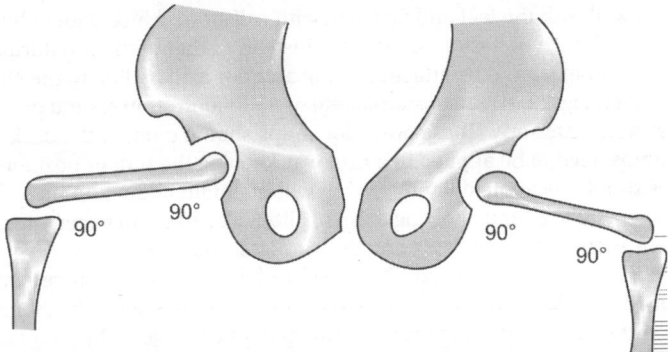

Fig. 22.8: 90°–90° position of hips and knees within Pavlik harness (shown by line diagram)

Treatment

The treatment of DDH should be started soon after birth. Most of the subluxatable hips if kept in abduction and flexion from the early part of neonatal period are corrected. The dislocatable and dislocated hips (Ortolani positive) even if treated early in abducted and flexed position may not be corrected in all the cases. Teratologic dislocated hips are not correctable without surgery.

The methods of abduction in flexion may be of different ways. Multiple diaper or Frejka pillow is the easiest way. Craig splint, although a rigid one keeps the hips in abduction and flexion allowing care of the perineum at the same time (Fig. 22.7). The method of dynamic holding of hips in abduction and flexion was felt by Arnold Pavlik, a Czechoslovakian orthopaedic surgeon. He reported treatment of 1912 patients in a harness devised by him in 1958 known as Pavlik harness, and used widely all over the world.[17] This is a dynamic way of holding the hip in abduction and flexion allowing movements of the hip within safe zone (30°-40° abduction and 90°—120° flexion). Beyond this amount of abduction, there is possibility of pressure on the medial circumflex artery, which supplies a major portion of the head, resulting in a possibility of avascular necrosis at a later date. The amount of flexion will depend upon the

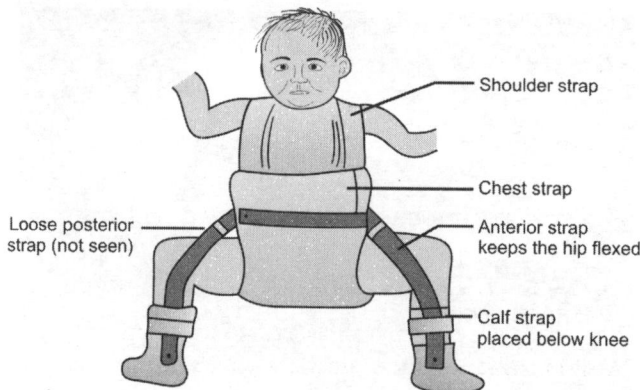

Fig. 22.9: Pavlik harness

tendency of the head to subluxate posteriorly and will be maximum up to 110° (Fig. 22.8). The stirrups of the harness should fit well with the feet and fastened with calf strap, which should be placed just below the knee to prevent occurrence of flexion of the knee instead of that of the hip during application. The anteromedial or flexion strap should be attached along anterior axillary line to the chest strap, which is placed at the nipple level (Fig. 22.9). The posterolateral or abduction strap should pass over the shoulder and fixed with chest strap anteriorly. These posterior straps should cross at the back over the scapulae. The anteromedial straps need to be applied in a firm way keeping the proper position of flexion but the posterolateral straps should be applied lightly, which will maintain abduction up to a maximum of 40° and will allow adduction up to a limit allowing a gap of about 8 to 10 cm between the knees.

The management with Pavlik harness though produces good results even with Barlow positive dislocatable or Ortolani positive dislocated hips, need to be monitored with care and precision. The harness is to be applied directly on the skin to avoid changing of clothes and to be maintained like that for the first four weeks. After this period, the time for bathing may be allowed. The straps should be properly applied and adjusted maintaining the correct position of the hip, which can be checked either by straight X-ray or ultrasonography.

As we are concerned in this monograph about the treatment of DDH in the neonatal period, further management will not be discussed except the treatment of complications as given below:

(i) If the child is irritable and reluctant to move the affected hip, the surgeon should search for inadequate reduction of the hip or femoral nerve palsy. Hyperflexion greater than 110°, specially in an obese baby, may cause irritation of the femoral nerve. Reduction of flexion helps amelioration of irritation of femoral nerve and the palsy in 3 weeks time, (ii) An ill fitting harness may cause medial instability of the knee because of excessive valgus force at the knee, (iii) Inferior or obturator dislocation occurs due to excessive flexion applied. A check X-ray helps to know the position and reduction of flexion corrects the position. If the dislocation persists, skin traction with about 2 to 3 lbs weight applied to both the lower limbs followed by closed reduction may help correction.

Pavlik harness is usually applied for about 2 months in most of the cases. Prolonged application may cause fixed anterior dislocation of the hip, which is a rare form of presentation of DDH in a virgin case. The cause is excessive abduction and external rotation of the hip. The femoral head is palpable in the groin in such a case. A lateral view usually help in the diagnosis. Failing which CT or MRI will delineate the head. Here again, skin traction with progressive flexion in slight abduction followed by closed reduction and plastering is the method to be followed. Persistence of acetabular dysplasia following treatment with Pavlik harness will be corrected usually be continued use of an abduction hip orthosis. If the hip is unstable, the treatment will be closed or open reduction and plastering.

Developmental Dysplasia of the Hip

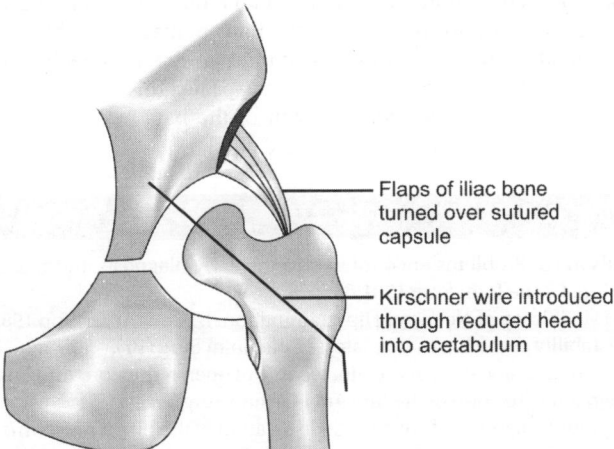

Fig. 22.10A: A modified open reduction of the hip dislocation showing flaps of iliac bone chiselled out and turned on the capsule in anteroposterior projection. The hip being fixed with a `K' wire after reduction

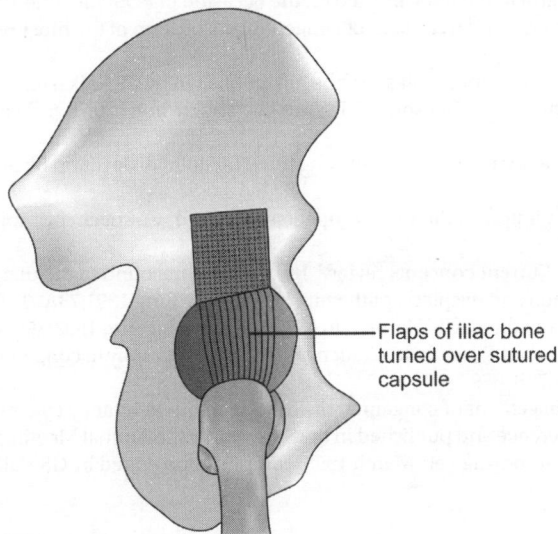

Fig. 22.10B: The same operation as in the Figure 22.10A shown from the lateral aspect

In a series of 41 infants with 42 unstable hips, treated by the author[18] only 12 infants with unilateral dislocation needed operative correction—a modified open reduction, where the sutured capsule of the hip, after excising the redundant part, is reinforced by flaps of iliac bone chiselled out and turned on the capsule (Figs 22.10A and B). These bony flaps with their lower ends attached, were sutured with the capsule with no. `O' vicryl suture for strengthening the capsule. This method is an attempt to prevent recurrence of dislocation, done at a period of growth of the baby when no corrective osteotomy is possible. The success rate is 83.34 per cent (ten in twelve hips).

REFERENCES

1. Mackenzie IG, Wilson JG. Problems encountered in the early diagnosis and management of congenital dislocation of the hip. J Bone Joint Surg 1981;63B: 38.
2. Tredwell SJ, Bell HM. Efficacy of Neonatal Hip examination. J. Pediatric Orthop 1981;1: 61-5.
3. Danielsson LG. Instability of the hip in neonates. J Bone Joint Surg (Br).
4. Howarth MB. Congenital dislocation of the hip: technic of open reduction, Ann Surg 1952;135:508.
5. LeDamaney P. Cogneneital luxation of the hip. Am J Orthop Surg 1914;11:541.
6. Andren L. Aetiology and diagnosis of congenital dislocation of the hip in newborns. Radiology 1961;1:89.
7. McKibbin B. Antomical Factors in the Stability of the Hip Joint in the Newborn. J Bone Joint Surg 1970;52-B (1):148-59,
8. Ilfeld FW, Westin WS, Makin M. Missed or developmental dislocation of the hip. Clin Orthop 1986;203: 276.
9. Ortolani M. Un Segno poco noto e sue importanza per la diagnosis precoce di preussasione congenita dellanca. Pe diatria, 1937;45:129, quoted by Dennis R. Wenger: Developmental Dysplasia of the hip, published by GS Kulkarni in the book printed on the occasion of POSI meeting 1998.
10. Barlow TG. Early diagnosis and treatment of congenital dislocation of the hip. J Bone Joint Surg 1962;44B: 292.
11. Dennis R Wenger. Development dysplasia of the hip, published by GS Kulkarni in POSI meeting 1998; p31.
12. Portinaro NMA, Mathews SJE, Benson MKD. The acetabular notch in hip displasia. J Bone Joint Surg 1994;76B: 271.
13. Graf R. New possibilities for the diagnosis of congenital hip joint dislocation by ultrasonography. J Pediatr Orthop 1983;3:354.
14. Tachdjian Mihran O. Clinical Pediatric Orthopedics. Stanford, Connecticut: Appleton and Lange; 1997. p.178.
15. Harcke HT, Kumar SJ. Current concepts review. The role of ultrasound in the diagnosis and management of congenital dislocation and dysplasia of the hip. J Bone Joint Surg 1991;73A: 622.
16. Suzuki S. Ultrasound and the Pavlik Harness in CDH. J Bone Joint Surg 1993;75B: 483.
17. Suzuki S. Kasahara Y, Futani T, Ushikubos Tsuchiye T. Ultrasonography in congenital dislocation of the hip. J Bone Joint Surg 1991;73B: 879.
18. De Mazumder N. Management of congenital dislocation of hip in infancy by a modified open reduction. Presented in the Conference and published in the Souvenir of the Annual Meeting of Pediatric Orthopedic Society of India, at Pune, during Feb-March 1998, compiled and edited by GS Kulkarni 71-75.

Chapter 23

Congenital Abduction Contracture of the Hip and Pelvic Obliquity

Keywords: Intrauterine malposture of the foetus in a first born baby is the cause – associated with dysplasia of the contralateral hip – passive stretching exercises in infancy is the key to correctiion.

INTRODUCTION

Since Weissman[1] first published this condition in 1954 reports have been made about it by Cozen[2] and Green and Griffin.[3] This congenital condition of abduction contracture of the hip and pelvic obliquity is frequently associated with dysplasia of the contralateral hip.[3] The cause of this condition is intrauterine malposture of the fetus, particularly when first-born.[4] Like windblown syndrome of the knees this condition is also called windblown syndrome of the hip.

CLINICAL AND RADIOLOGICAL FEATURES

The condition is detected clinically in a neonate by asymmetry of the gluteal folds and popliteal creases when looked from behind with the lower limbs held parallel to each other. The pelvis, raised on one side causing pelvic obliquity will be evident from the raised posterior superior iliac spine, gluteal and popliteal creases and apparent limb length inequality—the reason being abduction contracture of the hip of that side. The opposite adducted hip, which is often the left side was found to be dysplastic in 17 out of 18 children studied.[3] Other report[4] suggests the adducted hip to have no subluxation or dislocation as detected by ultrasonography, but may show congenital coxa vara or proximal femoral focal deficiency in AP view of straight X-ray.

The condition may be associated with other associates of malposition *in utero* like varus or valgus of feet, torticollis, plagiocephaly with or without cranial synostosis.

The degree of abduction contracture, due to tight iliotibial band is assessed by Ober test. Often there is associated external rotational contracture. The spine may be found scoliotic.

Differentiation from congenital dislocation of the hip is made by the presence of flexion deformity in pelvic obliquity as detected by Thomas test. The hip is fully extended or rather hyper-extended in congenital dislocation.

TREATMENT

The condition is easily treated early in infancy by passive stretching exercises of the abduction contracture four or five times daily, which give complete correction in about four weeks time. To prevent recurrence, further stretching exercises are necessary for an additional period of six to eight weeks.

PROGNOSIS

The prognosis of this condition is favourable except in some moderate variety, where, there is a tale-tell evidence of out-toeing gait when the child learns walking. Subluxation or dislocation when present needs correction as in the case of DDH.

REFERENCES

1. Weissman SL. Congenital Dysplasia of the Hip. Observations on the 'Normal' Joint in cases of unilaternal disease. J Bone Joint Surg 1954;36-B(3): 385-96.
2. Cozen Lewis. Some Evils of Fixed Abduction of the Hip. Clin Orthop 1968;57:203-11.
3. Green NF, Griffin PP. Hip Dysplasia Associated with Abduction Contracture of the Contralateral Hip. J Bone Joint Surg 1982;64-A(9):1273-81.
4. Tachdjian MO. Clinical Pediatric Orthopedics—The Art of Diagnosis and Principles of Management. Stamford CT:Appleton and Lange.pp.191-3.

Section 3: Vertebral Anomalies

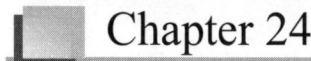

Chapter 24

Vertebral Agenesis, Fusions and the Fusion Defects

Keywords: Vertebral deformities at birth are due to agenesis, fusions and fusion defects of vertebrae-treatment is of neuromuscular defects which develop gradually.

To highlight the problems related to the absence or fusion of vertebrae, I would like to give a brief account of the embryological development of vertebral bodies, which will help better understanding of the pathology.

DEVELOPMENT OF VERTEBRAL BODIES

At about 5th and 6th week of intrauterine life mesenchyme condenses into segments to form sclerotome or somites. Subsequently these somites split. The upper part of one somite fuse with lower part of the upper somite to form a vertebral body. The central part of each somite incorporates a portion of the notochord, which forms the nucleus palposus, and together with the surrounding somite forms the intervertebral disc.

At different times of intra-uterine life three primary centres of ossification appear, one for each half of vertebral arch and one for the body of the vertebra. The centres of ossification of vertebral arches develop first in the upper cervical vertebrae at around the ninth week of intra-uterine life. The centers of ossification of the lower vertebral arches develop subsequently reaching the lower lumbar vertebrae at the end of the third month of gestation. The centres for the vertebral bodies also appear in the ninth antenatal week in the lower thoracic region with successive appearance at upper and lower levels ending at fourth intra-uterine month. During the first year of life the vertebral arches join together and ultimately begin to join with the vertebral bodies after the third year in the cervical region completing the process in the lower lumbar vertebrae in the sixth year.

The body of the odontoid process is ossified at birth and is connected with the body of the axis by cartilage. The apex of the odontoid process, which grows separately is also cartilaginous at birth.

How the Vertebral Bodies Look Like in X-ray at Birth?

The vertebral bodies almost oval in shape particularly in the lateral view with radiolucent area in the middle, which corresponds to penetration of vessels from both anterior and posterior aspects. The discs are thick showing a space, almost as wide as the vertebral body.

About the Stability of the Vertebral Column

To maintain an erect position, the vertebral column needs to be stable, yet maintaining various movements like flexion, extension, rotation and lateral flexion. The stability is maintained by both intrinsic and extrinsic means. The intrinsic stability is helped by the ligaments and muscles attached to the spinous processes, laminae and vertebral bodies along with the annulus fibrosus surrounding the intervertebral discs. The additional support of extrinsic stabilisation is by the thoracic cage with its intercostal muscles and ligaments along with the help of trunk muscles. What are the spinal defects or deformities observed in the neonatal period?

A. Spinal defects
   1. In spina bifida
      a. With normal development of spinal cord (closed variety)
      b. With abnormal development of spinal cord (open variety)
   2. In vertebral agenesis
   3. Congenital scoliosis.
B. Congenital abnormalities in the cervical spine
   1. Absence of a cervical vertebra or half of it
   2. Abnormalities of the odontoid process
   3. Absence or shortness of the neck
   4. Congenital postural and muscular torticollis.

Spinal Defects

Spina Bifida

Failure of fusion of two halves of the neural arch leads to spina bifida; which when associated with lesion in the skin, with protrusion of cord and meninges through it results in an open variety (spina bifida aperta). The other variety with intact skin is the closed one. The spinal cord may sometimes be undeveloped or dysplastic.

The cause of the condition is unknown. The incidence among orientals is not known; but it is higher among certain races, in first born children and in poor families.

Closed Spina Bifida

The association of certain conditions with spina bifida is well-known. Although a closed spina bifida is covered by intact skin, the clinical diagnosis is made from a dimple or a pigmented naevus or a faun's tail arising from skin. Associated dermoid cyst or a lipoma of nerve roots cause a bulge in the skin. Sometimes the condition is extended to agenesis of the sacrum or bifurcation of the cord by bony spur from posterior aspect of vertebral body, the condition is known as diastematomyelia. Herniation of the meninges without any neural elements in it, known as meningocele is on rare occasion may be an associated finding. X-ray confirms a gap in the neural arch or the presence of posterior bony projection from the vertebral body.

The condition when associated with neurological features, will need treatment. The neurological features occur long after neonatal period and is due to growth of the spinal cord with the growth of the body causing a traction effect on nerve roots, tethered at the site of defect. Only a meningocele needs treatment early in the neonatal period.

Open Spina Bifida

A neonate with a myelomeningocele protruding through the open skin at the lumbo-sacral region is a common finding. This is a meningeal sac which contains inside nerve roots and remnants of cord, often adherent to the sac. The condition is important from the point of view of contamination of infection into the central nervous system through the open skin and development of hydrocephalus on closure of the defect.

A new born baby with a postural defect or a classical deformity of club foot, claw toes, genu recurvatum or hip dislocation may be due to or associated with a translucent cystic lump in the mid-line of the back caused by myelomeningocele. When the deformities are due to the cause of the defect, these are from intra-uterine paralysis.

The initial management of such a case rests on a paediatric surgeon, who closes the defect as early as possible, preferably within 48 hours, to avoid a possible contamination of the CNS. This is simple skin closure after undermining of the skin preserving intact the neural structures. The closure of the skin will cause hydrocephalus, which may develop within a few days. The hydrocephalus is treated by paediatric or a neurosurgeon by a ventriculo-caval shunt using Spitz-Holter valve.

The patient is referred to an orthopaedic surgeon after the initial treatment is over, but should preferably be within the neonatal period to prevent the deformities going into a rigid variety. We often come across such cases with paralytic or isolated deformities, as mentioned earlier. The skin of the lower limbs, in such a case, is anaesthetic and the bones are fragile. The management starts with a straight X-ray of the spine and pelvis; and in case of genu recurvatum with X-ray of the knee. Muscle-nerve chart will detect the presence of paralysis. The correction of deformity will be gentle by repeated manipulation and strapping with occasional use of well padded splint to prevent ulceration on foot.

As the child grows the importance of management of paralysis with skin care and treatment of urinary problems intrigues a surgeon. Sometimes babies are born with neonatal kyphosis, which needs correction by osteotomy to close the skin defect. Excision of Kyphotic vertebrae allows fixation of two halves of the vertebra.

At a later age the child requires correction of deformities of his or her unbalanced paralytic limb. For flexion deformity of the hip elongation of psoas tendon with detachment of flexor muscles from ilium (Soutter) is the method of choice. In a balanced paralysis with flail limb all that is required is splintage to stabilise the limb. A dislocated hip mostly due to unbalanced paralysis needs psoas and adductor tenotomy prior to reduction by closed or open method with achievement of muscle balance by transplantation of psoas muscle from lesser trochanter to greater trochanter by either Mustard or Sharrard method. Failed reductions and older children need innominate or derotation varus osteotomy of femur or both simultaneously for the containment of the head of the femur into the acetabulum.

To allow the child to stand and walk the lower limb joints should be made suitable for use of a caliper. Surgery not only helps to correct the same but also helps to achieve balance between the muscles. The operations necessary to correct individual joints are not within the purview of this book.

VERTEBRAL AGENESIS

This congenital defect involving sacral and/or lumbar vertebrae with neural elements is evident at birth with associated genitourinary and lower intestinal anomalies. The first case was reported by Hohl in 1852.[1]

The vertebral defect may be an isolated one or may be associated with neural defect as studied by Smith.[1] The neural abnormality is a motor one without involvement of sensory nerves. The genetic factors causing both these defects in the early embryonic life are common ones as advocated by Lendon.[2]

Clinical Features

There are four different types of presentation at birth as reported by Renshaw.[3] The commonest being the partial bilaterally symmetrical sacral agenesis, the type 2 variety of Renshaw. The associated lesions here are foot deformities with or without subluxation of hip. The type 1 lesion is partial or total unilateral sacral agenesis with obliquity of lumbosacral joint and nonprogressing scoliosis is the rarest variety. The pelvic obliquity and the congenital scoliosis found in this type is associated with lower limb defect of the affected side. In the variable lumbar and complete sacral agenesis of type 3 lesions, the ilia articulate with the lowest lumbar vertebra, as evident in the prominent end of the lumbar vertebrae at the back and anteriorly rotated and narrowed pelvis with flattened buttocks. The neural element defect is very prominent in this variety causing paralytic foot deformities with genu recurvatum and dislocation of hips. The severe form or type four variety is the agenesis of sacrum and partially lumbar vertebrae. As the previous variety there is prominence of the lower lumbar spine in the back giving the appearance of a gibbus with a reduced distance between the ribs and the iliac crests. The stature of the baby is obviously short. The narrow and unstable pelvis is rotated anteriorly as in the type three variety with the hips and knees flexed with webbing of skin in the popliteal region. The hips are not dislocated and the foot deformities depend upon the paralytic muscles. All these varieties may be associated with visceral abnormalities, imperforate anus, duplication of ureter or urethral valves and incontinence of urine and faeces due to neurologic defect.

Treatment

In the neonatal period no definite management can be started except assessment of neuromuscular defect by muscle-nerve testing. For the cavus deformity with claw toes developed due to absence of second and third sacral motor roots the correction will be done at later age by plantar release, tendon transfer and if necessary telectomy. Assessment should always be made in the first few months after birth of activity in muscles suppled by the upper lumbar nerve roots, which remain as the only effective motor roots. The deformities in the hip, knee and foot develop as a result of over action of the healthy muscles over paralysed muscles. Therefore, the correction of the deformities requires severing or elongating the contracted muscular bands and reinforcement of paralysed muscles by healthy muscles. Dislocation of hip is corrected by closed or open-reduction as necessary. Sometimes the hips are left as dislocated when both the hips are affected. Internal rotation deformity of the thigh is corrected by psoas transfer to antero-lateral aspect of greater trochanter along with flexors release of hip from pelvis. Flexion and adduction in the hip are corrected by adductor release at the groin and psoas release medial to sartorius. The whole idea of doing these operations is to make the limb fit for an orthosis with a pelvic band with hip hinges. Sometimes the knee flexion deformity is not corrected by soft tissue release alone; bone shortening at the lower third femur with extension osteotomy will have to be done for proper fitting of an orthosis. These operations are done between six months and two years of age.

In the sacral and lumbar agenesis, absence of nerves necessitates in corrective varus-rotation osteotomy in the upper femur and amputation through the knee. In case of a flail limb with sensory loss in the foot sometimes subtrochanteric amputation is necessary between the ages of four and seven years. To bring stability to the pelvis along side the remaining lumbar vertebrae, vertebro-pelvic fusion is done at around six or seven years of age.

REFERENCES

1. Smith ED. Congenital Sacral Anomalies in Children, Australia and New Zealand. J Surg 1959;29:165-76.
2. Lendon.
3. Renshaw TS. Sacral agencies: A classification and review of twenty-three cases. J Bone Joint Surg 1978;60A:373.

Chapter 25

Congenital Scoliosis

Keywords: The underlying cause of congenital scoliosis is defective formation or segmentation of vertebral bodies – limiting growth of vertebral column in the convex side by epiphysiodesis or excision of hemivertebrae are important among the treatment protocol.

CONGENITAL SCOLIOSIS

The condition is sometimes diagnosed at birth. Diagnosis is made by X-ray of the spine, on a baby with slight lateral prominence on one side of the spinous process. The underlying cause may be congenital

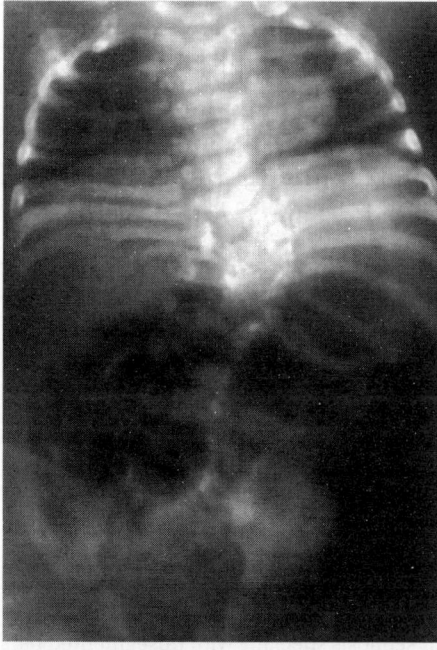

Fig. 25.1: Radiograph of congenital scoliosis in AP view showing hemivertebrae

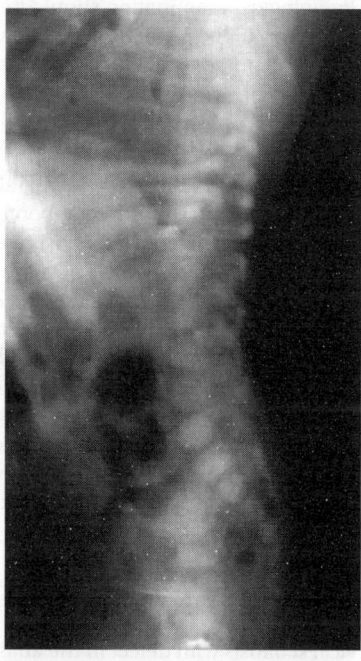

Fig. 25.2: The same patient as in Figure 25.1 showing lateral view

scoliosis involving a number of vertebrae. In others, a chest X-ray or straight X-ray of abdomen taken for some other cause, reveals scoliosis with congenital vertebral defects.

Cause and Diagnosis

The underlying cause is defective formation or segmentation of vertebral bodies. The pathological findings detected in the X-rays are wedged or hemivertebrae in case of defective formation (Figs 25.1 and 25.2) and unilateral unsegmented bar or in bilateral cases, vertebral fusion or block vertebrae are found due to defective segmentation.

The progress of scoliotic curve depends upon the nature of pathology. Multiple hemivertebrae or unilateral bars usually progress quickly resulting in a severe curve. During rapid spinal vertebral growth in the juveniles or in case of severe curve the deterioration is rapid. On the contrary a single hemivertebra or a slight curve formed by balanced hemivertebrae without unsegmented bars at a level close to each other usually does not progress.

If not detected early just after birth; congenital scoliosis is detected usually at a school going age. The growth of the scoliotic curve will be there as long as the growth of the body continues, with a spurt during puberty. The curve is well compensated in the cervico-thoracic region but is least compensated in the lumbo-sacral region. Thoracic lesions develop a deformity of the rib cage.

Clinical examination detects the level of the curve with associated kyphosis or lordosis when present.

Neurological examination should be done in all cases to detect any nerve deficit. Cranial nerves and upper limbs should be examined. Mild degree of hyprocephalus, Arnold-Chiari deformity or syringomyelia is sometimes found. Rib abnormalities like fusion, visceral anomalies like congenital heart disease and genitourinary abnormalities and musculo-skeletal abnormalities like Sprengel's shoulder, pectus carinatum or excavatum, club foot, congenital convex pes valgus, atrophy of a limb are sometimes associated findings.

Radiological examination should be in both AP and lateral views to detect the presence of kyphosis or lordosis or lumbosacral spondylolisthesis along with scoliosis. With the advent of MRI early detection of hydrocephalus, diastematomyelia has been possible.

Treatment

No treatment is possible in the neonatal period. Passive stretching exercises halt curve progression and postural active exercises improve poor posture. Conservative treatment with a plaster cast or a brace is necessary for congenital scoliosis having hemivertebrae with unsegmented bars, which generally progress from worse to worst. A curve of more than 50° usually does not benefit from conservative treatment and needs spinal fusion with or without instrumentation even at a young age. Convex growth arrest by hemiepiphysiodesis, both anteriorly and posteriorly is indicated. When there is potential growth in the concave side of the curve, specially in young children, excision of hemivertebrae is indicated for rigid curves in the lumbosacral area. Scoliosis with multiple hemivertebrae and balanced curve do not require treatment, except in some progressing variety.

Cervical lesions are sometimes associated with deficiencies of the atlas causing instability of the neck. Similarly cervico-thoracic scoliosis produces distortion of the shoulders and neck. Lumbar lesions are associated with pelvic obliquity and lordosis. All these lesions need spinal fusion with or without osteotomy, followed by bracing.

Prognosis

Cervical scoliosis with defect in the atlas and thoraco-lumbar scoliosis specially with unsegmented bars have worst prognosis followed by lumbo-sacral scoliosis because of lack of compensation from below and due to rapid development of irreducibility in the compensatory curve above.

Chapter 26

Klippel-Feil Syndrome

Keywords: Short and stiff neck with low hairline detected at birth–due to defect of fusion of cervical vertebrae at different or all levels–no treatment is possible in the neonatal period.

INTRODUCTION

This syndrome of short stiff neck with low posterior hairline is detected on many occasions just after birth.

ETIOLOGY

Failure of segmentation of the mesodermal element forming vertebral bodies during third to eighth week of intrauterine life causes this defect of fusion of cervical vertebra at different or all levels, atlanto-occipital fusion and cervical spina bifida. The cause is attributed to a subclavian artery supply deficiency.[1]

The first patient with this deformity, described by Klippel and Feil in 1912, died of renal failure.

CLINICAL FEATURES

The clinically evident short and stiff neck with low hairline is associated with facial asymmetry, pterygium colli or winged appearance of trapezius, elevation of the scapula, cervico-thoracic scoliosis, upper limb anomalies like syndactyly or supernummery digits. Congenital heart disease like interventricular septal defect, patent ductus arteriosus, patent foramen ovale, coarctation of aorta may be associated. Agenesis or an ectopic lung, absence of kidney, horse-shoe kidney, ectopic kidney, absence of ovary or vagina are difficult anomalies often associated with the condition.

Deafness, facial nerve palsy and spinal cord compression add misery to the defective child.

Radiological examination of the cervical spine should be done in AP and lateral in normal position, in flexion and in extension. Laminagram also helps when there is laminar fusion. Chest X-ray detects lung anomalies. Ultrasonography in young children detects visceral abnormalities. MRI and CT scan help in the detection of associated cord compression.

TREATMENT

No treatment is possible in the neonatal period. Passive stretching exercises help to maintain range of motion. Correction of torticollis and cervico-thoracic scoliosis improves the appearance of the child.

Improvement of webbed neck by plastic surgery and the short neck by partial thoracoplasty of the upper ribs has been suggested by some authors.

REFERENCE

1. Bouwes Bavinck JN, Weaver DD. Subclavian artery supply disruption sequence: Hypothesis of vascular etiology for Poland, Klippel-Foil and Moebius anomalies. Am J Med Genet 1986;23:903-18.

Chapter 27

Congenital Muscular Torticollis

Keywords: Torticollis present at birth–due to a swelling or tumour in the sternomastoid muscle due to an organising haematoma.

This asymmetric congenital deformity of the head and neck with unilateral contracture of the sternocleidomastoid is characterised by lateral flexion of the head towards the shoulder, the chin turning towards the opposite shoulder. The deformity is detected two weeks after birth when a swelling or tumour, as it is called, is detected in the muscle belly of sternomastoid near the sternal head. The condition is not genetic in origin. A variety of torticollis present at birth is postural one and is transient in nature.

The deformity is more common in girls and the right side is affected in 75 per cent of cases. Developmental dysplasia of hip is associated with the condition in about 20 per cent of cases.

CAUSE

The cause of contracture due to muscle fibrosis is hypothesized since Stromayer in 1838 first propounded birth injury to the sternomastoid muscle as the cause, as the condition was common in patients with history of difficult labour and also following breech and forceps deliveries. The supporters of the theory were favoured till Mikuliez advocated muscle ischaemia theory, supported by Adams. A link with obstetrical paralysis was found by Suzuki. More recently researchers advocated a venous occlusion theory due to malposition in uterus and compartment syndrome.[1]

CLINICAL FEATURES

Clinical appearance of a swelling, usually in the lower half of the sternomastoid muscle after about 10 days from birth, is very characteristic of this condition. Although the swelling is an organizing haematoma, yet it is popularly known as a sternomastoid tumour and disappears at around seven months time. The baby develops a contracture of the muscle after disappearance of the swelling leading to torticollis with lateral flexion towards the side of the tight muscle having the face and chin rotated towards the opposite side.

As the child grows the facial asymmetry and plagiocephaly, which may appear even in the neonatal period, will go on increasing. Sometimes the torticollis is unaccompanied by sternomastoid tumour. This condition is often associated with congenital club foot, developmental dysplasia of hip, internal torsion of tibia and metatarsus adduction.

Histological examination of the swelling shows degenerating muscle tissue with scattered cellular fibrous tissue in it, surrounded by disorganised endomysial sheath. Ultimate appearance, after a lapse of about six months, is mature fibrous tissue with contracted surrounding fibrous tissue.

Diagnosis in the neonatal period is difficult in the absence of a sternomastoid tumour. In that condition vertebral anomalies are often found, detected by X-ray.

TREATMENT

Torticollis is corrected in the neonatal period by gentle manipulative stretching by the mother in the opposite direction of the deformity, usually in prone position to reduce muscle spasm. In case of a painful tumour, rest to the neck is given by placing pillows by the side of the neck. Manipulation is started as the pain subsides. Usually the torticollis is corrected in three to six months time. Residual deformity is corrected by gradual correction in a harness. Gross facial asymmetry is of bad prognostic significance and the torticollis and asymmetry of face remain even after correction. In very obstinate cases in older children unipolar tenotomy of clavicular head and 'Z' plasty of sternal head of sternomastoid with excision of contracted deep fascia is done; failure to produce correction will need division of upper attachment to mastoid, popularly known as bipolar sternomastoid tenotomy. The operation gives best results between one and four years of age.

Early operation in the neonatal period is avoided as this produces ugly scar.

REFERENCE

1. Davids JR, Wenger D, Mubarak SJ. Congenital muscular torticollis: Sequelae of intrauterine or perinatal compartment syndrome. J Pediatr Orthop 1993;13:141.

Section 4: Upper Limb and Shoulder Girdle Anomalies

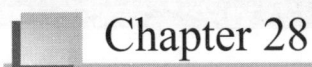
Chapter 28

Congenital High Scapula (Sprengel's Shoulder)

Keywords: Restricted shoulder movements with highly placed scapula–due to imperfect descent of the shoulder girdle in the intrauterine life.

This rare deformity is suspected at birth when the shoulder movements are limited and the scapula is placed at a higher level. The condition was first described by Eulenberg in 1836 but it was Sprengel,[1] who described many more cases and hence the deformity goes by his name. The deformity is three times more common among girls.

ETIOLOGY

Although the condition is detected at birth, it progresses with growth and becomes fully evident in early adolescence. The deformity results from imperfect descent of the shoulder girdle in the intrauterine life at around 9th to 12th week.

CLINICAL FEATURES

The fully evident deformity is a highly placed scapula, either unilateral or bilateral. The position of scapula may be as high as the level of upper cervical vertebrae almost reaching the occiput. The condition is associated with congenital fusion of cervical vertebrae.

DIAGNOSIS

The diagnosis is made by highly placed scapula, with the presence of a fibrous to bony mass attaching the scapula with the vertebrae, often clearly palpable, known as omovertebral mass. The shoulder movements are restricted, limiting abduction caused by the absence of normal rotation of scapula. The clavicle in the affected side is tilted upwards. The fully grown deformity of adolescence may be divided into four grades, needing different types of surgical correction, will not be described here. However, a straight X-ray is necessary to know the position of scapula and the presence of an omovertebral mass. In the early infancy a harness is all that is necessary for the correction of the deformity when a bony omovertebral mass is absent. The presence of the mass will necessitate in surgery at a later date for the correction of the deformity.

REFERENCE

1. Sprengel O. Die angeborene Verschiebung des Schulterllates nach oben. Arch Klin Chir 1891; 42: 545, quoted by Tachdjian MO: Clinical Pediatric Orthopedics, The art of Diagnosis and Principles of Management, Stamford CT: Appleton and Lange; pp.282-9.

Chapter 29

Congenital Pseudoarthrosis of the Clavicle

> **Keywords:** Nontender swelling lateral to middle of right clavicle mostly-producing pseudoarthrosis with painless motiion-treated by surgery betwen 1 and 3 years of age-bony union is achieved quickly.

This condition is detected at birth or in the neonatal period as a nontender swelling situated slightly lateral to the middle of the right clavicle having a variable degree of painless motion at that site on passive movement. The left clavicle is rarely affected, when the condition is associated with dextrocardia. Very rarely both clavicles are affected.

ETIOLOGY

The cause is failure of fusion of the two centres of enchondral ossification from which the clavicle develops; normally the fusion occurring at seventh week of gestation. The cause may also be defective normal ossification of the precartilaginous bridge, which connects the acromial and sternal ossification centres of the clavicle.

Further suggestions are made as to the cause of pseudoarthrosis. An exaggerated pulsation of the highly placed right subclavian artery is the cause of increased incidence of pseudoarthrosis on the right side. In a dextrocardiac baby the incidence is on the left side which further substantiates the theory.

As to the higher position of the subclavian artery on the right side is the observation of vertically oriented and abnormally high position of first and second ribs on the right side in cases of pseudoarthrosis of right clavicle.

There is very rare report of familial incidence.

CLINICAL FINDINGS

The swelling in the clavicle develops due to enlarged opposing ends of the clavicular fragments, the medial or the sternal fragment being larger than the lateral one and is placed slightly higher than the other due to pull of the sternomastoid muscle. The outer acromial fragment is inferiorly placed because of the weight of the upper limb too. As mentioned earlier there is painless motion of variable degree at the site of pseudoarthrosis on passive movements of the arm of the affected side.

DIAGNOSIS

The condition is diagnosed by clinical findings as described before and to be differentiated from fracture clavicle, neurofibromatosis, and cleidocranial dysostosis.

In fracture of the clavicle there will be a history of birth trauma and the baby will show pseudoparalysis of the upper limb of the affected side. There will be tenderness at the site of fracture, which will subside as the union progresses and the swelling at the fracture site will subside with the consolidation of the fracture union, which usually takes place in three to six months.

In case of neurofibromatosis the bone ends are attenuated instead of swollen and there will be other stigmata of neurofibromatosis.

The condition cannot be mistaken with cleidocranial dysostosis as the latter is often bilateral with absence of whole or major portion of the clavicles without the presence of any swelling at the site of the calvicles. Other associated skeletal deformities with cleidocranial dysostosis in the neonatal period are bossing of the skull, small facial bones, widening of the symphysis pubis (difficult to diagnose in the neonatal period, as this is normally found then).

TREATMENT

No treatment is recommended in the neonatal period. Surgery is advised between one and three years of age. The bone ends are excised, curetted and fixed internally with a threaded Kirschner wire. Autogenous iliac grafts are put around the site of pseudoarthrosis. The bony union is achieved quickly with the improvement in the strength of the shoulder girdle.

Chapter 30
Cleidocranial Dysostosis and Congenital Absence of the Pectoral Muscles

Keywords: Absence of clavicle in its middle or outer third - rarely evident at birth - autosomal dominant - radiograph shows deficiency or absence of clavicle - no specific treatment is suggested as the disability is minimum.

CLEIDOCRANIAL DYSOSTOSIS

This developmental affection of the skeleton is characterised by the absence of clavicle in its third—either in the middle or in its outer third, occasionally in its inner third or rarely in its entirety. The condition affects the bones formed in membrane like the clavicle, the cranium and the pelvis. Some of the bones preformed in cartilage like the short tubular bones of the hands and feet are also affected. The cause of the condition is unknown but inheritance as an autosomal dominant trait has been suggested.

Clinical Findings

The condition is rarely evident at birth. The diagnosis is made in early infancy or in childhood. A baby with a large brachycephalic head and bossing of frontal, parietal and occipital bones with wideset eyes in his small retrognathic face should be looked for absence of part or whole of clavicle either unilaterally or mostly bilaterally. Because of the hypoplastic nature of sternomastoid and anterior fibres of deltoid muscle in a narrow chest and absent clavicle the shoulders can be brought nearly together anteriorly. In the pelvis the space between the symphysis pubis is enlarged. The dentition is often delayed and abnormal.

Radiodiagnosis

Radiographically the deficiency or absence of clavicle is evident either unilaterally or bilaterally. The skull shows enlarged anterior fontanelle with multiple wormian bones. In the pelvis the innominate bones show delayed ossification with a wide symphysis pubis. Manubrium sterni is poorly developed and the spine shows spina bifida occulta in the thoracic and lumbar region due to failure of ossification and closure of the lamina. Later in the childhood the hands and feet show delayed ossification of the carpal and tarsal bones with short phalanges and large second metacarpals.

Treatment

No specific treatment is suggested as the disability is minimum.

CONGENITAL ABSENCE OF THE PECTORAL MUSCLES

This absence of pectoral muscles is evident in a newborn baby and the nipple over the absent muscle is often atrophic. Often syndactyly and microdactyly are associated with when the condition is known as Poland's syndrome.[1]

REFERENCE

1. Ireland DCR, Takayama N, Flatt A. Poland's syndrome. J Bone Joint Surg 1976;58A:52.

Chapter 31
Congenital Radioulnar Synostosis and Congenital Synostosis of the Elbow

Keywords: Three different types according to the presence or absence of the radial head and the nature of radioulnar coalition of bony or ligamentons nature – results are poor after separatiion of synostosis. Congenital synostosis of the elbow is treated by rotation osteotomy and bone lengthening where necessary.

CONGENITAL RADIOULNAR SYNOSTOSIS

The deformity is present at birth. The mother complains of loss of rotation of one or both the forearms, the latter being fixed in a position of neutral rotation to hyperpronation.

Etiology

The deformity occurs due to failure of longitudinal segmentation of the mesodermal tissue forming the cartilaginous anlage of the radius and ulna. There is an arrest in the development with either fusion of the radius and ulna at its upper end by the ossified mesodermal tissue between them or the mesodermal tissue forming the interosseous ligament thickens and binds together both the bones of the forearm preventing rotation.

Classification

The condition is classified in three different types according to the presence or absence of the radial head and the nature of radioulnar coalition—bony or ligamentous. In type I the radial head is absent with complete fusion of the radius and ulna at its upper end—the headless type. In some of the type I cases the radial head though present, does not show any motion as the head with the upper radius is completely fused with the ulna (Fig. 31.1). In type II the radial head is dislocated posteriorly and the part of the upper radius below that is synostosed to the ulna. In type III the interosseous ligament is short and thick, which prevents rotational movements of the forearm. There is no bony fusion in this type.

Diagnosis

The condition is diagnosed in the neonatal period from the mother's complain of a flexed attitude of the elbow, either unilateral or bilateral with varying amount of atrophy of the forearm, the latter being placed in pronation. The restriction in supination movement of the forearm is a diagnostic finding. In

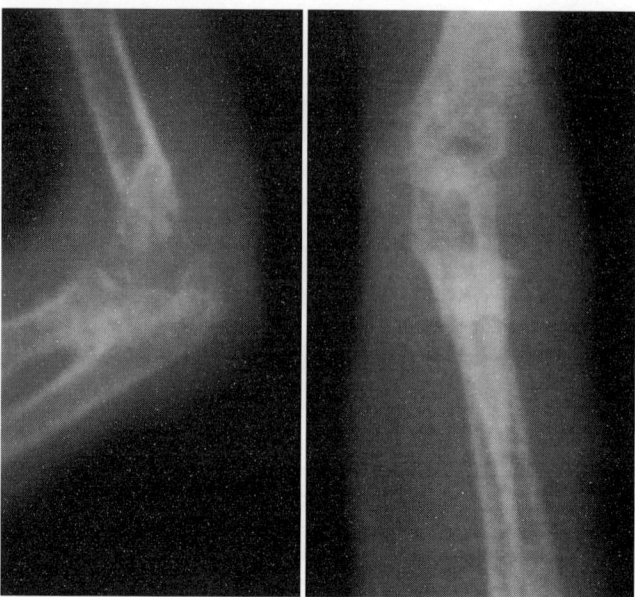

Fig. 31.1: Radiographs (AP and lateral views) of congenital radioulnar synostosis showing fusion of radius and ulna at their upper ends

the type I variety where the head of the radius is completely fused with the ulna or absent, a dimple may be found at the site where the normally positioned radial head would have been. Various types of difficulties in daily activities in an older child are due to limitation of supination movement, the amount of movement being slightly less than the full range to a complete absence. The wrist and shoulder joints have normal movements. The shoulder may show excessive rotational movements in an older child because of difficulties caused by the limitation of supination of the forearm.

Treatment

No attempt for the separation of the synostosis should be made at any age as the results are poor. The rotational movements can be achieved by osteotomy of the radius at its middle third; the forearm is placed after the correction in neutral position. Where the amount of rotational correction needed is more than 45°, both the radius and ulna are osteotomised. In bilateral cases the dominant forearm should be placed in 30° to 45° pronation and the other forearm in 10° to 30° supination.

CONGENITAL SYNOSTOSIS OF THE ELBOW

A baby presenting at birth with stiff elbow having the forearm fixed in varying degrees of flexion and pronation associated with moderate to severe atrophy and shortening of the upper limb is a sufferer from congenital synostosis of the elbow. The condition may be unilateral or bilateral in occurrence, often in association with some other congenital anomaly of the upper limb. When the ulna is absent the synostosis occurs between the humerus and the radius.

Two important points are to be considered in the management of the condition. The first is a rotation osteotomy of the hyperpronated single bone of the forearm, when the condition is presented like that, to achieve an improved functional position of the hand. And the second is lengthening of the bones of the upper limb when the shortening is severe, making the condition a demanding one for treatment.

Chapter 32

Radial Club Hand and Congenital Longitudinal Deficiency of the Ulna

Keywords: Radial club hand – typed according to the partial or complete absence of radius – treatment at birth by splintage – corrective surgery at the age of three and a half years when carpal bones start to displace volar and radially. Congential longitudinal deficiency of ulna is very rare – to have a functioning forearm rdius needs a derotatiion osteotomy – a short ulna needs elongation surgically.

RADIAL CLUB HAND DEFORMITY

The radial club hand deformity has been described under different names since 1733.[1] It is found at birth associated with other congenital deformities. The basic deformity of radial club hand is absence or hypoplasia of the radius resulting in bowing of the forearm radially and deviation of the hand towards the radial side, giving a prominence of the lower end of the ulna as a stump. The thumb is mostly absent or a floating one. This is a congenital longitudinal deficiency of the radius and so the forearm is short in length. The obvious clinical appearance and the conspicuous absence of part or whole of the radius is radiographically present at birth.

The condition is not very common and the frequency of occurrence is one in 30000 births.[2] The mortality rate of infants with radial defects at birth as reported by Warkany[3] is very high and the surviving children with the defect have a high mortality rate upto the age of twenty.

Etiology

Thirty-five children with radial club hand as reviewed by Wynne-Davies[4] showed no genetic pattern in the occurrence of the deformity tracing the families to at least the third degree relatives.

In a large series of sixty-eight babies with 117 radial club hand deformities,[1] twenty-six of the sixty-eight mothers were found to have ingested thalidomide and fourteen had taken some unidentified medium during the early months of pregnancy. Twenty-eight mothers had no significant history and the pregnancies were normal.

Of the various theories suggested as the cause of radial club hand the one propounded by Saunders[5] is most tenable. His work on chick embryos suggested that damage to the apical ectoderm on the anterior aspect of the developing limb bud leads to the deformity.

Anatomy of the Radial Club Hand

As suggested by different authors the condition is not a simple preaxial deficiency of the upper limb but also shows abnormalities of muscles, nerves and joints. The thumb is either absent or floating. The

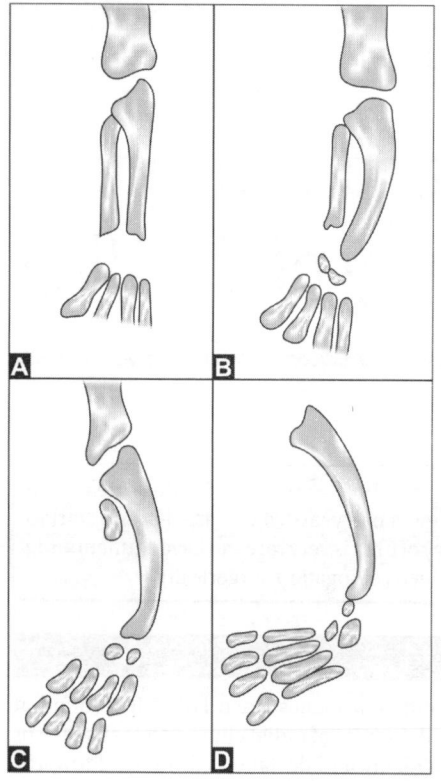

Figs 32.1A to D: Types of radial club hand-type I and II showing short radius, type III showing complete absence of the distal and middle part of the radius and type IV depicting absence of the radius

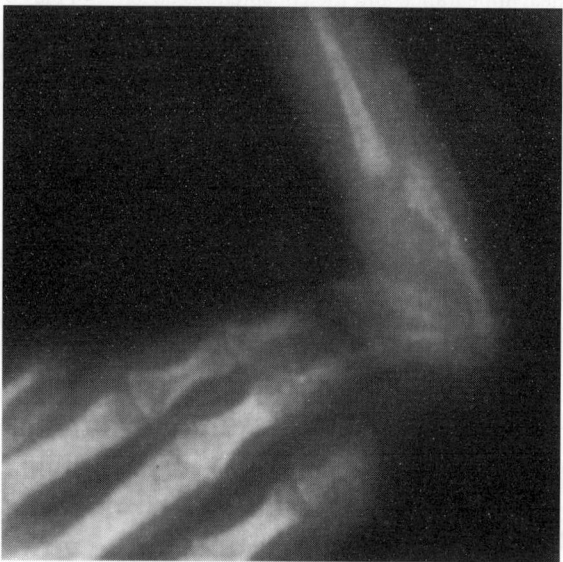

Fig. 32.2: Radiograph showing radial club hand

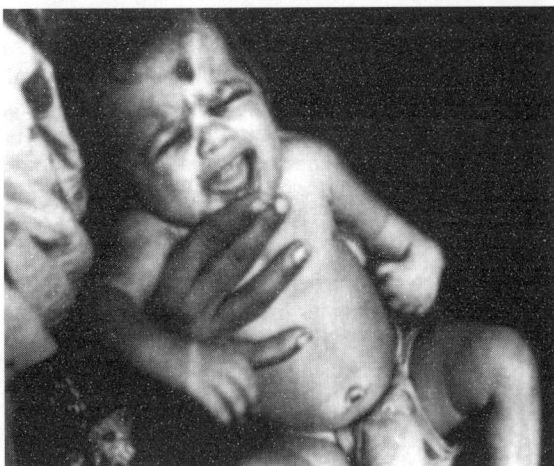

Fig. 32.3: Clinical photograph of radial club hand of the left side showing diminished length of the forearm

bowing of the ulna is rare in babies at birth but develops as a secondary deformity due to soft tissue contracture at the deformed wrist. The radius may be hypoplastic where the distal radial epiphyseal plate is deficient with delay in the ossification of the center of the lower epiphysis developing into a short radius (type A) shown as type I and II in Figures 32.1A to D; the distal and middle part of the radius may be completely absent (type B) shown as type III in Figure 32.1; and complete absence of the radius (type C), shown as type IV in Figures 32.1A and in a radiograph (Fig. 32.2). The radial side of the carpal bones is nearly always deficient. There is absence or deficiency of the muscles arising from the common extensor origin specially the extensor carpi radialis longus and brevis along with volar muscle like flexor digitorum profundus of the index finger. All these lead to a dysfunction of wrist joint motion from minor stiffness to almost no motion and poor function of the digits of the radial side than those of the ulnar side. In an untreated radial club hand the wrist is unstable due to radial and volar displacement of the carpal bones due mainly to the unopposed action of the wrist flexor and partly by the finger flexors, particularly the flexor digitorum superficialis.

There are some striking differences in the growth of the forearm and arm in children having radial club hand (Fig. 32.3). The ulna is often shorter in length and compared to the length of the humerus of that limb it may of the ratio of 3:2 or 2:1. This is because the distal ulnar epiphysis appears later in radial club hand and also closes earlier than in normal children.[6] As said earlier the motion in the wrist joint is jeopardised due to the asymmetrical growth of the muscles in the deformed radial club hand, so is the movement in the digital joints. While the metacarpophalangeal joints have excessive hyperextension and limited flexion, the proximal interphalangeal joints will have fixed flexion deformities with skin webbing in some. The radiographs of these joints do not show any change in the joint outline and so, the cause of the limited motion is extra-articular. The range of motion of the distal interphalangeal joint is increased on active movements, more on the ulnar than on the radial side. Often the elbow is fixed in extension in some of the patients with radial club hand.

Associated Anomalies

Involvement of many other organs in congenital anomalies is quite common with radial club hand. Blood dyscrasia like Fanconi pancytopenia and thrombocytopenia are often associated with absence of the radius known as TAR syndrome. In a study of 54 children of Lamb's series Gillespie[7] found 26 patients whose mothers consumed thalidomide during pregnancy and other group of nonthalidomide or idiopathic group of 28 patients. In the thalidomide group limb deficiency in other bones was found in 7 of the 26 patients, where limb deficiency of other bones was absent in the non-thalidomide group. Visceral anomalies of various types was found in both types of patients. Congenital and idiopathic scoliosis and patent ductus arteriosus were common anomalies in both the groups. Other anomalies like imperforate anus, oesophageal atrasia, ventricular septal defect, tetralogy of Falot, coarctation of aorta, renal agenesis, pedunculated encephalocele with communicating hydrocephalus were some of them. Atrial septal defect with radial club hand (Holt-Oram syndrome) was not found by Gillespie.[7]

Treatment

The treatment should be started from birth. The deformed hand should be put to a corrected position by a splint. The deformity is easily correctable after birth with a simple splint. In difficult cases the correction is obtained gradually by a ratchet-type splint. The splint is worn even six months after correction of the deformity by surgery. When the child starts using his hands, the splint is worn only at night. This is necessary to prevent contracture. The only other conservative treatment is mobilisation of a stiff elbow, when that is present.

The question of corrective surgery arises at about the age of three and a half years when the carpal bones start to gradually displace in a radial and volar direction. Various methods of surgical corrections have been described in the literature. The procedures when analysed were found to be of four different methods of correction. The oldest method of correction was soft tissue release and ulnar osteotomy. Different types of ulnar osteotomies were described since Hoffa[8] first described it in 1890. Sayre,[9] Bardenheuer and Romano also described different types of ulnar osteotomies, but they were not very effective. Replacement of the radius by a bone graft was practised by Albee, Ryerson, Starr and Riorda but these also were not successful as alignment could not be maintained by them.

Then came the most practised procedure of centralization of carpal bones under the ulna. If the ulna is curved it may require correction by osteotomy. As to the time of surgery opinions differ. But most authors like Mercer, Tachdjian and Salter recommend early surgery. Those authors in favour of early surgery advised maintenance of correction during growth of the baby to achieve a good functioning hand. Here the question arises whether the baby would have the same function if left untreated, as raised by Lloyd-Roberts and other surgeons. Lamb,[1] who showed good functional results in a large series of 117 radial club hand deformities in sixty-eight patients, showed favourable results even when the elbow was stiff by mobilizing it. He strongly recommended the presence of active elbow flexion of at least 90 degrees prior to centralisation of carpal bones. He has shown no significant increase in the natural shortening of the forearm following correction, which strongly disfavours the point against surgery. The function of the wrist was not jeopardised following surgery in his series, which was contrary to that observed by many others. Lamb took the help of tendon transfers in some of this surgically treated cases to ensure better function of the wrist. In type A the simplest variety, the radius is only lengthened.

The method of surgical correction of centralisation of carpal bones will not be described in the present book, but the role of pollicisation or transposition of the index finger to take the function of the thumb, after the correction of the wrist deformity needs mentioning. Transposition of the index finger is possible if its muscles and the structure of the joints are sufficiently normal to take the function of the thumb. According to Lamb[1] the operation improves the function of the hand to a considerable extent and recommends this procedure in both unilateral and bilateral cases and not in only the dominant hand of the bilateral affection, as has been suggested by many. The operation is always done after the benefit of centralisation of the carpal bones is well enjoyed by the child and hence the procedure of pollicisation is done between one and thirteen years, the average time being seven years.[1]

CONGENITAL LONGITUDINAL DEFICIENCY OF THE ULNA

Unlike longitudinal deficiency of radius this deformity is very rare. The ulnar clubbing with which the baby presents is obvious at birth. The forearm is flexed in hyperpronation with frequently present ankylosis of the elbow.

To make a functioning forearm the radius needs a derotation osteotomy to make the forearm 30° supinated. A short ulna is better treated by elongation following any of the available technique with orthofix or Ilizarov method.

REFERENCES

1. Lamb DW. Radial club hand J Bone Joint Surg 1977;59A:1-13.
2. Birch-Jenson Arne. Congenital deformities of the upper extremities. Translated from the Danish by Elisabeth Aagenson. Copenhagen theses, Odense, Andelsbogtrykkeriet, 1949, quoted by Lamb DW.
3. Warkany Josef. Congenital malformations. Notes and comments. Chicago, Year Book Medical Publishers, 1971, quoted by Lamb DW.
4. Wynne-Davies R. Hritable Disorders in Orthopedic Practice. London, Blackwell Scientific Publications 1973.
5. Saunders JW Jr. The Proximo-Distal sequence of origin of the parts of the chick wing and the role of the ectoderm. J Exp Zool 1948;108: 363-403, quoted by Lamb DW.
6. Heikel HVA. Aplasia and hypoplasia of the radius. Studies on 64 cases and on epiphyseal transplantation in rabbits with the imitated defect. Acta Orthop. Scandinavica, Supplementum 1959;39.
7. Gillespie WJ. Personal communication, 1973, quoted by Lamb DW.
8. Hoffa Albert. Lehrbuch der orthopoidischen chirungic, ed 4, Stuttgard, Ferdinand Enke, 1092, 557, quoted by Lamb DW.
9. Syre RH. A contribution to the study of the club hand. Trans Am Orthop Assn, 1893;6:208-16, quoted by Lamb DW.

Chapter 33

Hand and Finger Affections Present at Birth

Keywords: Various hand and finger deformities presenting at birth – embryologic defect – hand reduction syndrome is a distinct variety – the deformities may be part of congenital syndrome or an isolated variety.

Various types of deformities involving hand and fingers present at birth are due to failure of differentiation of adjacent fingers or simple duplication of a single embryologic bud or due to hyper or hypo or no growth of an embryologic bud. The reduction of hand as a whole is a distinct entity. The deformities of hand and fingers may be relatively common varieties of syndactyly or polydactyly or deficiency of thumb or miscellaneous finger affections often with flexion deformities (Fig. 33.1)[1]. The deformities may be part of a congenital syndrome or an isolated variety. Often we come across congenital band syndrome which is commoner in lower limbs than in the upper ones. The incidence of hypertrophy of one or two fingers or a congenital trigger thumb is not very common. Of the twenty five per cent of trigger thumb present at birth, fifty per cent are cured automatically by 12 months time. Here lies the importance of detection of the deformity at birth.

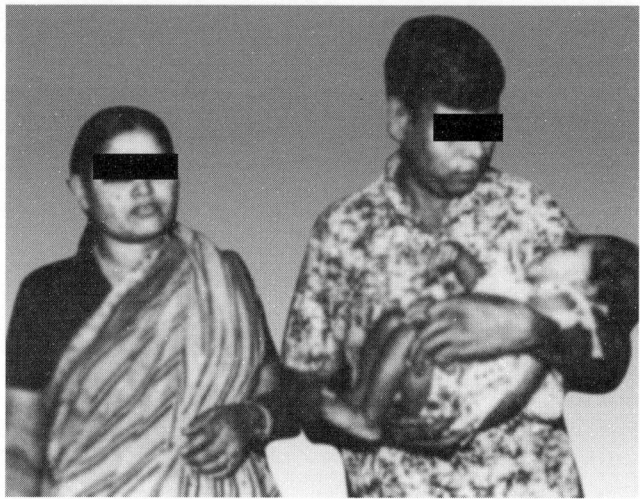

Fig. 33.1: Flexion deformities of fingers shown in the photograph of the father and the baby in his lap

SYNDACTYLY

Syndactyly or fusion of adjacent fingers occurs due to failure of differentiation between adjoining fingers in the embryonic life. It is the most common congenital anomaly of the hand present at birth with an incidence of one in every 2000 live births. Boys are affected more than the girls in the ratio of 2:1. The familial incidence is not very common, which is about one-fifth of total occurrences.

Types of Syndactyly

The syndactylism may be a simple one with involvement of skin only to a complex variety where the bones of the adjacent fingers are fused with sometimes joining of tendons and nerves. When the fusion occurs throughout the length of the digit upto the tip of the finger, the syndactylism is a complete one. The bony fusion is detected by radiography.

The middle and ring finger syndactyly is the commonest (60%) as against syndactyly between ring and little fingers with an incidence of 27 per cent. Rarest of all syndactyly is between thumb and index finger as the thumb develops earlier than other fingers. The condition may happen as part of a syndrome like Apert syndrome where all the fingers are involved (mitten hand). Often the fingers are short with deficiency of the long bones also. The condition may be part of Poland syndrome when the ipsilateral pectoral muscles are absent or associated with constriction bands, known as Streeter syndrome. Sometimes a polydactyly presents with syndactyly.

Treatment

Although the treatment of this condition is mainly surgical separation, the fingers joined together at the tip needs passive extension, as active extension is difficult in these cases. The passive stretching should be started in the neonatal period to prevent development of contracture of fingers.

As regards time for surgery, early operation at around 18 months of age is indicated in condition like Apert syndrome, as the development of fingers is retarded if the fingers are left unseparated. In other cases, as single entity, the time for surgery is delayed upto the age of five years.

In multiple finger involvement the prominent finger should be given more importance. As skin flaps grow faster than split thickness graft with the general growth and development, the important finger like the middle one should be separated from the syndactyly with the ring finger and the skin coverage on the medial side of the middle finger should be made with the palmar and dorsal flaps from the ring finger. Split thickness grafts are used to cover the defects on the ring finger. The techniques of various methods will not be described as these are not within the purview of this book.

POLYDACTYLY

Supernumerary digit due to duplication of a single embryologic bud gives rise to polydactylism and is easily diagnosed at birth. The extra digit is commonly lateral to thumb (preaxial type) or medial to the little finger (postaxial type) or along ring, middle or index finger (central type). The condition may be associated with polydactyly of toes, with congenital anomalies like duplication of the breast or nipple.

Incidence

Postaxial polydactyly is commoner than preaxial variety. The incidence of the former in blacks is 1 in 300, ten times more than in the whites. The incidence of preaxial polydactyly has no racial variation and is 0.08 per 1000. When the postaxial polydactyly is part of a syndrome in whites, it is an isolated one in blacks. Hence the hereditary predisposition is autosomal recessive in whites but dominant in blacks.

Types

The extra finger may be constituted of soft tissues only hanging from the outer aspects of thumb or little finger, either of equal size as that of normal finger or hypoplastic. When the duplicated finger consists of bones—the phalanges inside may articulate with a common metacarpal or a duplicated one. The last variety forms a separate digit having mostly common nerve and blood supply and tendinous disposition.

The duplication of the thumb has been critically analysed and divided into seven different types by Wassel.[1] He has described the types according to the variation of duplication from distal to proximal. The type I is very rare, only 2 per cent of all occurrences, where the distal phalanx is bifid. In type II the distal phalanx is duplicated and occurs in 15 per cent. Similarly in type III the distal phalanx is duplicated, articulating with a bifid proximal phalanx in 6 per cent cases; whereas in the next variety or type IV the proximal and distal phalanges are both duplicated and articulate with a common metacarpal. This fourth variety is the commonest, i.e. 43 per cent. In type V duplicated proximal and distal phalanges articulate with a bifid first metacarpal occurring in 10 per cent cases. Type VI is again rare, i.e. 4 per cent where duplicated phalanges and metacarpals articulate with a common carpal bone. The last variety, type VII shows duplication of the entire thumb, which is triphalangeal, occurring in 20 per cent cases.

Treatment

As the thumb has got some important functions to perform the excision of a duplicated thumb needs proper care to maintain alignment, stability, vascular supply and motor control. A hypoplastic duplicated finger can be removed easily at any time after the birth of the baby. But a fully duplicated finger with its three phalanges, metacarpal and soft tissue components needs to be excised by proper surgery at 6 to 12 months of age of the baby.

CONGENITAL LONGITUDINAL DEFICIENCY OF THE THUMB

As in other longitudinal deficiency of a bone the thumb deficiency may vary from a floating thumb to simple hypoplasia to complete absence. An obvious deformity like a floating thumb or an absence of thumb is detectable at birth. The condition may be an isolated one or part of a syndrome. In a floating thumb the metacarpal is partially or completely absent. A hypoplastic thumb contains metacarpals and phalanges within but sometimes is devoid of any tendon.

Longitudinal Deficiency of Thumb as Part of a Syndrome

In Carpenter's or Rubinstein-Taybi syndrome hypoplastic thumb is found in association with brachydactyly.

In the presence of longitudinal deficiency of other bones like radius the condition is part of Fanconi or Holt-Oram syndrome.

The first metacarpal in some type of longitudinal deficiency of the thumb is often short and broad as a part of Cornelia de Lange syndrome.

In the affections of both hand and feet with shortening of thumb and great toe the condition may be myositis ossificans progressiva.

Treatment

A floating thumb without any metacarpal or a hypoplastic thumb without any tendon has very little function and better excised. This may then be treated like absence of thumb with pollicization of index finger. To achieve abduction and opposition movement, transfer of tendon is done to the pollicized index finger.

In a hypoplastic thumb with proper functions of the metacarpophalangeal and interphalangeal joints, the web between the thumb and index finger is deepened for better functioning of the thumb.

Web Contracture between Thumb and Index Finger

The contracture or syndactyly between thumb and index finger may occur with a hypoplastic thumb or as a part of syndactyly between other fingers, where the thumb is normal in size. As mentioned before the latter condition is rare as the thumb develops earlier than other fingers.

As the function of the hand is very much jeopardised due to contracture between the thumb and the index finger, the separation between the metacarpals of two fingers is achieved by lengthening the web between the two through Z-plasty.

MISCELLANEOUS FINGER DEFORMITIES

Finger deformities detected at birth are clinodactyly as found in Down syndrome and camptodactyly. The Kirner deformity is usually detected at about puberty. One report shows two cases might have their presence at birth.[2]

Clinodactyly

Clinodactyly is hereditary deformity commonly of the little finger, which is curved mediolaterally at the proximal or distal interphalangeal joint with the tip of the finger turned towards the ring finger. Sometimes bilateral, the deformity is of autosomal dominant inheritance. Surgical correction is required for cosmetic purpose and where the deformity is severe enough to interfere with normal hand function. The correction is by closing wedge osteotomy.

Camptodactyly

Camptodactyly is also an affection of the little finger mostly and ring finger rarely. This is a flexion deformity. The bending here is commonly at the proximal interphalangeal joint and sometimes at the distal interphalangeal joint. Correction by extension - dorsal wedge osteotomy is rarely necessary at it does not improve motion in the affected joint.

Kirner Deformity

The Kirner deformity is mostly bilateral one, where the terminal phalanx of the little finger is deviated laterally and palmar wards, appearing spontaneously at about puberty, as mentioned before. Rarely does this deformity appear at birth.[1] This is of autosomal dominant inheritance, where family history is rarely found. Kauffmann and Taillard[3] noted through histopathology a definite lysis between the diaphysis and the epiphysis of the terminal phalanx as the cause of the deformity. The correction of the deformity is rarely necessary.

CONGENITAL CLASPED THUMB

This deformity is diagnosed at birth from the characteristic position of the acutely flexed thumb, lying across the palm of the hand—the flexion adduction deformity of the thumb.

The condition is caused by hypoplasia or aplasia of the extensor pollicis brevis.

The clinical difference between this deformity and the congenital trigger thumb is positional—the former is the flexed attitude at the metacarpophalangeal joint and the latter is due to flexion at the interphalangeal joint.

The treatment is splintage from the neonatal period into extension-abduction. In stubborn or resistant cases Z-plasty is done to elongate the webbed skin. Sometimes after soft tissue release and obtaining extension-abduction of the thumb, the skin is covered by a rotation flap from dorsum and a full-thickness skin graft.

CONGENITAL TRIGGER THUMB

This condition when present at birth is easily diagnosed from the flexed attitude of the thumb at the interphalangeal joint, which appears like a trigger. When passively released from the flexed attitude the extended position is achieved with a triggering effect.

Incidence

The deformity is found at birth in 25 per cent cases, with a bilateral occurrence of 50 per cent. The rest 75 per cent cases develop later in childhood at around two years of age, when the bilateral involvement is only 25 per cent.

Etiopathology

The cause is stenosing effect produced by tendovaginitis of the flexor pollicis longus tendon. The cause of tendovaginitis is not known. However familial incidence is found sometimes. There is no genetic cause.

Pathologically a nodule develops on flexor pollicis longus tendon proximal to a stenosing constriction of the fibrous flexor sheath of the tendon. Histology of the sheath shows nonspecific chronic inflammation.

Differential Diagnosis

An osteoma of the proximal phalanx or metacarpal of the thumb mimics the condition clinically. The presence of flexed attitude of the thumb in most of the cases and radiography differentiate the conditions.

Treatment

As spontaneous recovery occurs in about one-third cases in the congenital group, conservative treatment of passive stretching of the thumb is followed several times a day. If the deformity persists, surgical correction is done at around two to three years age of the child. The procedure is a simple release of the sheath of the flexor pollicis longus under general anaesthesia at the site of the nodule on the tendon. Portions of the tendon sheath from the two sides of the longitudinal release are removed to prevent adhesion of the sheath with the tendon and for proper gliding movement of the tendon. The digital nerve to the thumb should be taken care of during surgery.

HAND-REDUCTION MALFORMATIONS

The malformation of hand-reduction constitutes a large heterogenous group having different radiologic anatomy with the presence or absence of associated malformations and the presence or absence of genetic cause. The report of Robert T Pilarski and his associates[4] of 61 different cases is worth mentioning. 15 of 61 hand-reductions, i.e. one-fourth of the total cases resulted from abnormalities of single genes of which the vast majority were autosomal dominant and more than one-third (21 of 61) were part of multiple malformation syndrome.

Pilarski et al followed the diagnostic classification presented by Tamtamy and McKusick.[5] 23 of 61 hand-reductions were terminal transverse defects, 14 were radial defects; eight were ulnar defects of which five were isolated, two were femoral-fibular-ulnar syndrome and one of Pallister syndrome[6] (a pleiotropic dominant mutation affecting skeletal, sexual and apocrine-mammary development); one isolated radioulnar defect; seven had split foot and split hand of which one had Karsch-Neugebauer syndrome; and eight had isolated split hand with terminal transverse defect in two. In the Karsch-Neugebauer syndrome in one of the 61 cases, a 46 year old woman and three of her six children had both split foot and split hand and congenital nystagmus, said to be a single gene dominant disorder.

In hand-reduction malformations as part of a syndrome, the secondary features like heart disease in Holt-Oram syndrome, visual impairment in Karch-Neugebauer syndrome, though initially seem to be less obvious may ultimately be of serious health problem.

Family history is also of importance in patients with hand-reduction malformation as 13 patients in Pilarski's series had positive family background.

REFERENCES

1. Wassel HD. The results of surgery for polydactyly of the thumb. A review. Clin Orthop 1969;64:175.
2. Dykes RG. Kirner's deformity of the little finger. J Bone Joint Surg 1978;60B: 58.
3. Kauffmann HJ, Taillard WF. Bilateral incurving of the terminal phalanges of the fifth fingers. American Journal of Roentgenology, Radium Therapy and Nuclear Medicine 1961;86:490-5.
4. Pilarski RT, Pauli RM, Engber WD. Hand-Reduction Malformations: Genetic and Syndromic Analysis. Journal of Ped Orthop 1985;5: 274-80.
5. Tamtamy SA, Mckusick VA. The genetics of hand malformations. Birth Defects 1978;14: 35.
6. Pallister PD, Herrmann J, Opitz JM. Studies of malformation syndromes in man XXXXII : A peiotropic dominatn mutation affecting skeletal, sexual and apocrine-mammary development. Birth defects 1976;12:247.

Section 5: Neonatal Infections

Chapter 34

Neonatal Osteomyelitis

Keywords: Osteomyelitis in neonates—may be part of septic arthritis or not—pseudoparalysis and/or local swelling is the feature—causative bacteria *Staphylococcus aureus* and B-haemolytic *Streptococcus* mostly—antibiotic therapy after blood culture—surgical drainage may be necessary.

NEONATAL OSTEOMYELITIS

Osteomyelitis in neonates, although not very common, differs significantly from osteomyelitis occurring in older children. The condition may either manifest as a very benign one in an apparently normal infant, as it happens in the majority, or this may appear as an incident in a disease process like septicaemia.[1-5] However, the term 'benign' relates to the clinical presentation only and not the real picture of the disease, which may produce serious complications producing permanent disability.[3,5]

Controversies remain as to the predisposing cause of the disease. When 22 of 35 infants showed predisposing factors like prematurity, skin or umbilical sepsis, delivery by cesarean section, jaundice, pneumonia and meningitis, as described by two authors,[6] absence of history of maternal obstetrical complication or umbilical sepsis was predominant in another series.[7]

The blood supply to the epiphysis in the neonate is a direct continuation of the diaphyseal blood supply, which crosses the epiphyseal plate[2] till the epiphyseal growth plate develops to act as a barrier of diaphyseal blood supply. The transepiphyseal vessels disappear at about the age of one year or a little later. So, acute osteomyelitis is often accompanied with acute septic arthritis in neonates and in early infancy.

Clinical Features

Ninety-five per cent of babies have either pseudoparalysis and/or local swelling. Abnormal posture is also a feature in many causing pain on passive movements of the affected limb. In order of site of affections, the hip comes first, followed by distal femur, proximal humerus, proximal tibia and other sites.[6] Involvement of multiple sites has been reported in 40 per cent patients.

Associated with Septic Arthritis

Bacteriology

Seventy two per cent growth of *Staphylococcus aureus* has been reported in 74 per cent culturally positive patients in a significant number of 34 affected neonates, having no gram-negative infection in the series.

Where B-hemolytic *Streptococcus* was detected in 28 per cent (7 patients) of the above series consisting of group A in one patient and group B in six; other series[7] emphasized the importance of group B B-hemolytic streptococcal infection in 69 percent infants with osteomyelitis and/or septic arthritis in less than two months of age. Infection with gram negative rods (*Haemophilus influenzae*) has been reported by some authors.

Pathology

An initial involvement shows soft tissue oedema of superficial tissues rapidly turning into spotty areas of destruction and absorption of bone trabeculae due to local hyperaemia. When the infection spread to regional cortex, subperiosteal abscess forms. As the blood supply to metaphysis of long bones in neonate communicates with the blood supply to the epiphysis, the infective process extends to the epiphysis resulting in destruction of the epiphysis in many cases causing major growth disturbance. The spread of infection is rapid due to poor inflammatory reaction and immature immune response in neonates resulting in gross destruction of metaphysis and epiphysis and also affection of multiple sites.

Radiographic Changes in Straight X-ray

The early cases show soft tissue changes as revealed by oedema in fatty planes of muscles, which in one to two weeks time is replaced by spotty irregular areas of rarefaction in the metaphysis and epiphysis due to destruction and absorption of bone trabeculae and due to local hyperaemia. Subperiosteal abscess when found, is revealed in ultrasonography.

Metaphyseal rarefaction and periosteal reaction are two characteristic features (Figs 34.1 and 34.2). Where septic arthritis sets in (Figs 34.3A and B) subluxation or dislocation of joints develop quickly (Fig. 34.4). As the involvement of hip is quite common, it has been suggested that every septicemic neonate should have the X-ray of the pelvis to exclude occult sepsis of the hip.

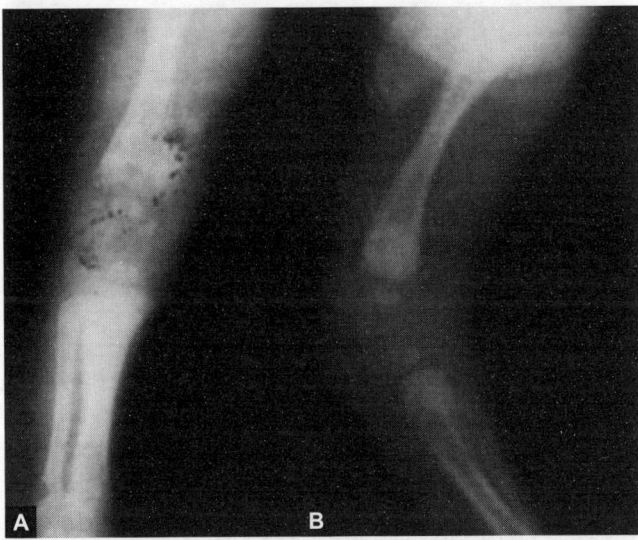

Figs 34.1A and B: Neonatal osteomyelitis—metaphyseal rarefaction and periosteal reaction shown in lower end of femur and upper end of tibia

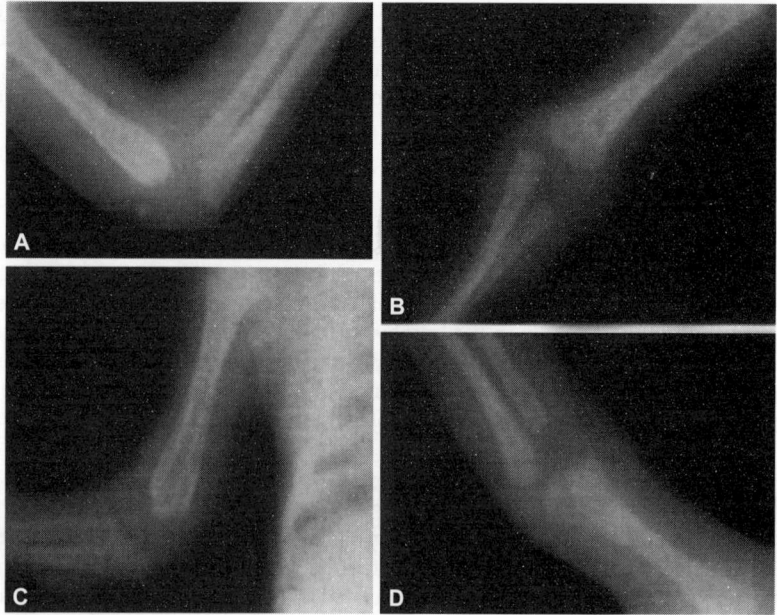

Figs 34.2A to D: Neonatal osteomyelitis—metaphyseal rarefaction and periosteal reaction shown in lower end of humerus and upper ends of radius and ulna

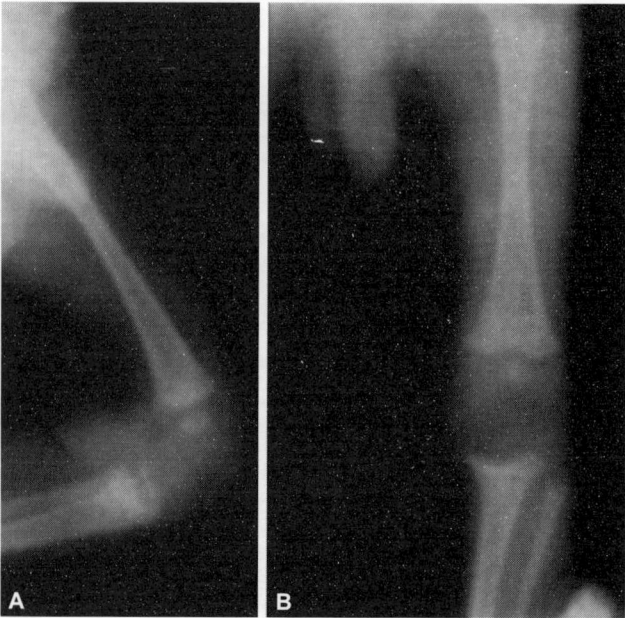

Figs 34.3A and B : Neonatal osteomyelitis showing established septic arthritis in the knee joint with scalloped upper epiphysis of tibia and distended capsule producing a huge soft tissue swelling

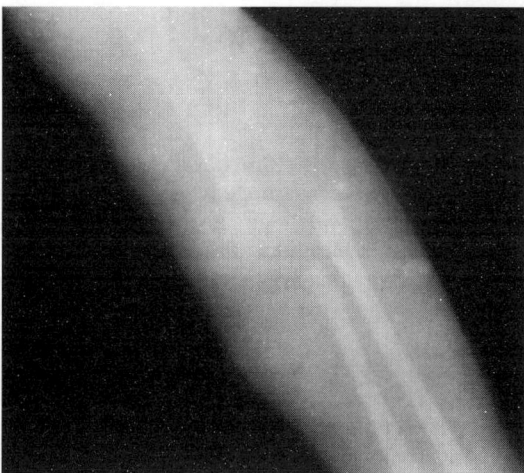

Fig. 34.4: Neonatal osteomyelitis showing hugely distended lower end of arm and upper end of forearm having the elbow dislocated medially

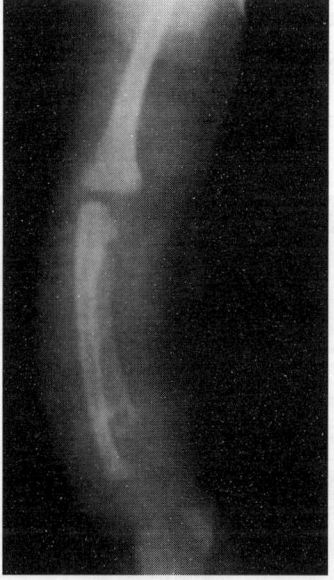

Fig. 34.5: Neonatal osteomyelitis—a sequel shown in the diminished size of the radius from damage to growth plate

Diagnosis

Clinical features of swelling and pseudoparalysis help in the diagnosis. A high sedimentation rate, positive culture and radiographic features confirm the diagnosis. White cell count is not a very important feature in diagnosis. Isotope scanning with Technetium-99 is usually unreliable in the neonatal period,[8,9] except in cases of multiple sites of involvement. The importance of early diagnosis has been emphasised by many authors.[6,10-13]

Prognosis

Culturally *Staphylococcus aureus* is a sinister point in prognosis[9,11-14] specially when cloxacillin resistant. Different results have been published by different authors. When 68 per cent excellent results have been claimed due to immediate surgical drainage, with adequate antibiotic cover and appropriate splintage by two authors,[6] high failure rate was claimed by others,[9,14] specially when the predominant involvement was septic arthritis of hip from upper femoral involvement. Prematurity has also been incriminated for bad prognosis. An immature immune response has been shown in premature babies.[15]

Management

Adequate antibiotic therapy after blood culture is the main stay in treatment. Cloxacillin (200 mgm/kg/day) is usually used as the antibiotic of choice in *Staphylococcus aureus* infections and is continued for a minimum period of 48 hours by intravenous route. Cefotaxim or Gentamycin is used in B haemolytic streptococcal infection. Polyantibiotic therapy has become a common practice in recent years.

Rest to the part by splintage, specially in older children with involvement of joints, is followed in each and every patient. The hip joint which is commonly affected, is treated in abduction splintage till such time the capital epiphysis is well within the acetabulum and has shown signs of regeneration of the involved epiphysis. In spite of adequate splintage, the femoral epiphysis may remain deformed with or without dislocation.

Aspiration is of no use. Surgery is undertaken for the drainage of pus, specially when the joint is involved. Only occasional cases without involvement of joint require no surgery. The necrotic material is sent for histopathological examination to exclude necrotic neoplasm.

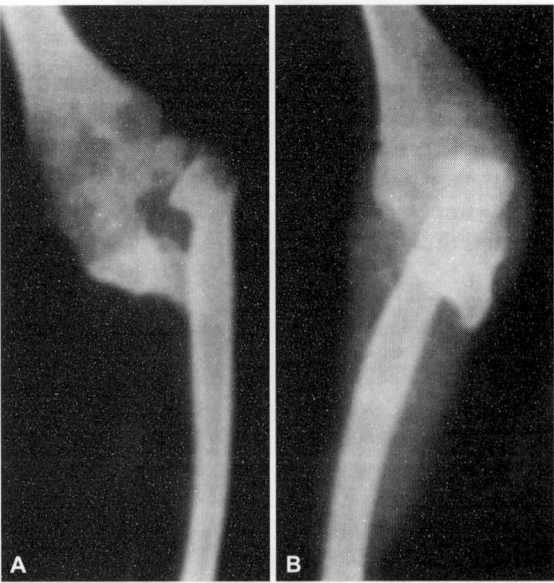

Figs 34.6A and B: Neonatal osteomyelitis—the forearm is deformed due to necrosis of the lower two-third of the ulna from osteomyelitis in the neonatal period

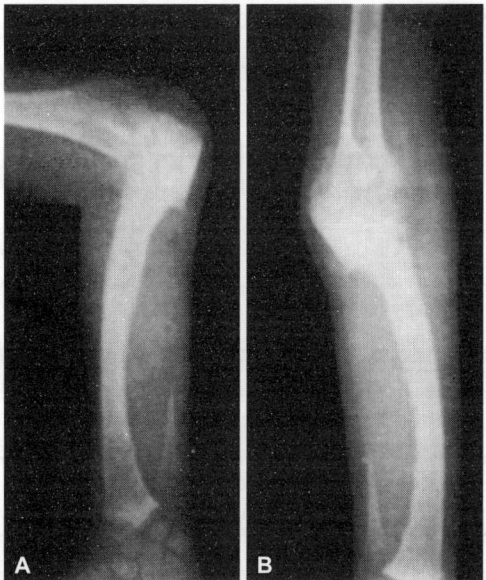

Figs 34.7A and B: The same patient as in Figure 34.6 salvaged by fusing the lower radius with ulna making an one-bone forearm

Complications

Injury to growth plate may lead to total destruction with subluxation of joint. The damage to growth plate may cause inequal or asymmetrical growth of the bones of the limbs (Fig. 34.5) with progressive deformity. A deformity of forearm due to necrosis of the lower two-third of the ulna from neonatal osteomyelitis shown in (Figs 34.6A and B) has been corrected by the author by excising the upper end of the radius and fusing the lower radius with ulna making an one-bone forearm (Figs 34.7A and B).

REFERENCES

1. Greengard (1946). Quoted from Kundsen C.J.M. and Hoffman E.G. J. Bone Joint Surg 1990;72B: 846-51.
2. Hutter CG Jr. New concept of osteomyclitis in the newborn infant J Pediatr 1948;32:522-79.
3. Thomson J, Lewis IC. Osteomyclitis in newborn. Arch Dis Child 1950.pp.273-9.
4. Potter CMC. Osteomyclitis in the newborn. J Bone Joint Surg 1954;36B:578-83.
5. Dennison WM. Haematogenous osteitis in the newborn. Lancet 1955;ii: 474-6.
6. Kundsen CJM, Hoffman EB. J Bone Joint Surg 1990;72B: 846-51.
7. Vidyasagar D. Text Book of Neonatology, Interprint 1988;36.
8. Ash JM, Gilday DL. The futility of bone scanning in neonatal osteomyclitis J Nucl Med 1980;21:417-20.
9. Berdahl S, Ekengren K, Eriksson M. Neonatal Haematogenous osteomyclitis. J Pediatr Orthop 1985;5: 564-8.
10. Blanche DW. Osteomyclitis in infants. J Bone Joint Surg 1952;34A:71-85.
11. Obletz BE. Acute suppurative arthritis of the hip in the neonatal period. J Bone Joint Surg 1960;42A:23-30.
12. Weissberg, Smith and Smith (1974). Quoted from Kundsen CJM, Hoffman EB J Bone Joint Surg 1990;72B: 846-51.
13. Lloyd-Roberts GC. Suppurative arthritis of infancy. J Bone Joint Surg 1960;42-B;706-20.
14. Hallel T, Salvati EA. Septic arthritis of the hip in infancy: End result study: Clin Orthop 1978;132:115-28.
15. Kuo KN, Lloyd-Roberts GC, Orme IM, Soothill JF. Immuno deficiency and infantile tone and joint infection. Arch Dis Child 1975;50:51-6.

Chapter 35

Acute Psoas Abscess in a Newborn Infant

Keywords: A rare case of psoas abscess in a neonate – not recorded before – diagnosis was made from clinical findings and increased WBC count – operative findings clinched the diagnosis.

ACUTE PSOAS ABSCESS

The youngest baby, a 31 day-old boy, who suffered from acute psoas abscess was reported by Zych and McCollough[1] in 1985. He was born after a normal delivery and his birth weight was 2.81 Kg. He suffered from moderate diarrhoea one week before he was first seen but his appetite was good. Prior to this he suffered from coryza and cough.

On admission the patient had slight dehydration, the rectal temperature was 36.8°C and the pulse was 140/min and regular. The leucocyte count was 11400/cmm and the blood urea nitrogen was 45 mgm percent. The chest X-ray showed evidence of bronchitis. The patient was treated with intravenous fluid in the intensive care unit and the investigations for infection began. He was shifted to general ward as his condition improved.

The condition of the baby deteriorated on the third day when he was put on intravenous penicillin and gentamycin pending the report of blood culture. The blood count went up to 17400/cmm, but the patient still had no temperature. The patient did not improve and a routine right femoral venepuncture on the 5th day could show inadvertently some purulent material from the right inguinal area. The material showed gram-positive cocci on the smear and the culture report was pending.

On the 5th day of admission the patient was still afebrile, but the white blood cell count went up further to 20000/cmm. There was swelling around the right groin, buttock and the upper thigh with 40° flexed attitude in right hip. The hip on passive movements was painful, specially on extension. The spine showed slight increase in lordosis. The radiography of the right hip showed only soft tissue swelling around the hip and the upper thigh region. The aspiration of the right hip did not reveal any fluid.

The right hip was explored by a posterior surgical approach keeping in mind a provisional diagnosis of septic arthritis of the right hip. The hip was completely free from any infection but the proximal femur area anteriorly revealed purulent material from the anterior hip region which helped in changing the diagnosis to a psoas abscess. Through anterior iliofemoral approach the psoas muscle was exposed which showed purulent material under its covering fascia and the other areas were dry. The pus was drained and the material sent for culture. After thorough irrigation and debridement of the affected muscle a Penrose drain was left at that site. Closure of the skin incision was made loosely.

There were both clinical and pathological improvement. The blood count came down to 15200/cmm. The pus culture showed *Staphylococcus aureus* which was similar to the blood culture sent from the intensive care unit. The baby was put to intravenous cloxacillin (200 mgm/kg/day) for 3 weeks. The patient was discharged from the hospital on the 35th day. The four years follow-up revealed an asymptomatic child with normal gait. The radiography of the pelvis and spine showed normal appearance.

The diagnostic point in this case was increased white blood cell count and the clinical findings. But the accuracy of the diagnosis was obtained from the operative findings. This is a rare case as the occurrence of psoas abscess in a neonate was not recorded before.

REFERENCE

1. Zych SA, McCollough NC. Acute psoas abscess in a newborn infant - a case report, Journal of Pediatric Orthopedics 1985;5:89.

Section 6: Miscellaneous Conditions

Chapter 36

Mucolipidoses

> **Keywords:** Coarseness of facial appearance in a generally retarded baby–vertebral and long bone changes in the X-ray–a storage disease of mucolipids in body tissues.

Spranger and Wiedemann[1] categorised mucolipidoses intermediate between mucopolysaccharidosis and sphingolipidosis. Excessive storage of mucolipids in a number of body tissues leads to a variety of disorders manifest at birth showing signs of skeletal changes. These are gangliosidosis type I and Mucolipidosis II (I-cell disease).

GANGLIOSIDOSIS TYPE I

This extremely rare disease mimics features of Hurler syndrome and presents at birth. Retardation of general development with coarseness of facial appearance are characteristic of this syndrome. Improper feeding due to poor suckling, feeble cry, enlargement of tongue, hepatosplenomegaly and stiffness of joints with cherry-red macular spot on ophthalmoscopy in 50 per cent cases, absence of mucopolysaccharide in the urine and excessive periosteal bone formation, nontender enlargement of epiphyseal parts of joints due to cartilaginous hypertrophy are diagnostic features of this syndrome.

This inherited disease is of autosomal recessive type and most of the babies with this disease die of respiratory insufficiency in the first few weeks of life and those who survive suffer from spastic quadriplegia, blindness and deafness and seldom cross second year of life.

The enzyme b galactosidase is specifically deficient in this disease in many tissues like brain, kidney, liver, spleen, skin, leucocytes, urine and in cultured fibroblasts.

Radiographically there are changes in the vertebrae and long bones. The anteroposterior diameter of vertebral bodies is reduced with hook-like appearance of lower thoracic and upper lumbar spine. There is excessive periosteal bone formation unlike Hurler syndrome. Naturally, the long bones, the ribs and the clavicle are wide.

Mucopolysaccharidosis and sphingolipidosis manifest long after birth and hence will not be discussed here.

MUCOLIPIDOSIS II (I-CELL DISEASE)

The clinical and radiological features are like gangliosidosis type I. The signs are manifested at birth. The inheritance is of autosomal recessive type but no specific enzyme defect is found. However, there is deficiency of a number of lysosomal enzymes and electron microscopy shows membrane bound inclusions within lysosomes in cultured fibroblasts.[2]

The affected babies die of cardiac and respiratory failure and rarely live beyond early childhood.

REFERENCES

1. Spranger J, Wiedemann HR. The genetic mucolipidoses. Diagnosis and differential diagnosis. Humangenetik 1970;9:113.
2. Hanai J, Leny J, O'Brien JS. Ultrastructure of cultured fibroblasts in I-cell disease. Amer J Diseas Child 1971;122:34.

Chapter 37

Neonatal Tetanus

Keywords: Neonatal tenanus develops from unbilical sepsis by *Clostridium tetani*–death rate is improved due to immunisation of pregnant mothers–neutralisatiion of tetanus by ATS and TIG is the key to treatment.

NEONATAL TETANUS

Tetanus as the cause of death in the neonates is of significance even today. About 6.5 per cent death in infancy in India is from tetanus 2.3 to 2.8 lacs infants die of neonatal tetanus every year.

Etiology

The causative organism *Clostridium tetani* gets entrance into the neonates body through contamination of the umbilical cord and causes tetanus after an incubation period of 3 to 14 days. The death rate from neonatal tetanus has come down significantly specially among the urban population because of immunisation of pregnant mothers.

The condition is diagnosed from unexplained excessive cry with refusal of feeds and apathy shown by the neonate. Spasm of neck muscles leads to opening of the mouth to a small extent. The attempt to open the mouth fully to feed the baby causes reflex spasm of the masseter muscles leading to lock jaw. The face shows a typical appearance known as 'risus sardonicus'; there is difficulty in swallowing, generalised rigidity of the neonates body amounting to opisthotonos and breathing difficulty.

Treatment

The treatment should be started as early as possible. The tetanus toxin needs neutralization by antitetanus serum (ATS) and tetanus immune globulin (TIG). The dose of ATS is 750 to 5000 units by IV or IM route and of TIG 250 units IV. The umbilical cord stump should be cleaned with hydrogen peroxide and spirit. Parenteral crystalline penicillin is administered 1-2 lac units per kg per day for 1 to 2 weeks. Spasm of muscles is controlled by 2 to 5 mgm of diazepam alternately with chlorpromazine 2 mgm per kg per dose by slow IV route every 2 to 4 hours.

Muscle relaxant like methocarbamol (50-75 mgm/kg/day) is administered by IV route twice daily or mephenesin 30-120 mgm/kg per dose is given orally hourly.

As the baby suffers from breathing difficulty, care of the airway is very important with the administration of oxygen. The baby's nutrition will have to be maintained and proper nursing care is necessary to prevent complications.

Chapter 38

Syndromes with Skeletal Problems, Present at Birth

Keywords: Of many syndromes, Down and Marfan syndromes are commoner.

DOWN SYNDROME

In babies with Down syndrome 95 per cent have three free-standing copies of chromosome 21, 1 per cent are mosaic with some normal cells and 4 per cent have a translocation involving chromosome 21.

Presenting Features

A flat face with slanting eyes, outer canthus above the uvea of the inner canthus, small rounded dysplastic ears with poorly formed antihelix and small ear lobule are characteristics of facial appearance of a Down syndrome baby at birth.[1] The presence of simian crease in palm is characteristic. Later in childhood with the flat face the nasal bridge becomes flat, the palate becomes high arched, the teeth erupts smaller than normal, the occiput becomes flat, the hands become short and broad with short fifth finger. The mental development is retarded.

A Down syndrome baby suffers from extreme hypotonia, lack of an abnormal Moro reflex and hyperextensibility at birth. The X-ray of pelvis shows dysplasia with prominence of anterior superior iliac spine, flat acetabula with indentation in the region of posterior superior iliac spine.

Diagnosis

Women about 35 years of age have increased risk of trisomy 21 and need to be diagnosed prenatally by amniocentesis or chorionic villus sampling.

Foetal chromosome analysis is another reliable method to diagnose foetal Down syndrome.

In women less than 35 years of age prenatal serum testing helps as a screening method.

Differential Diagnosis

Like Down syndrome, trisomies of chromosome 18 or 13 are also relatively frequent with manifestation of congenital anomalies and mental retardation.

Atlantoaxial instability and occipito-atlantal instability in 10 to 25 per cent cases, imperforate anus, leukaemia, lymphocytic thyroiditis, pulmonary vascular disease, abnormalities in eyes like Mongoloid slant of palpebral fissures, epicanthus, dacryostenosis, blepheritis, Brushfield spots of iris, peripheral thinning of iris stroma, keratoconus and corneal hydrops, cataract, high refractive errors, strabismus, nystagmus, increased vessels at disc are some of the features present in this syndrome.

Patients with Down syndrome have 10 to 30 times risk of developing leukaemia than general population. Neonates and infants with Down syndrome may suffer from a syndrome of transient myeloproliferation mimicking congenital leukaemia.

MARFAN'S SYNDROME

Tall stature of a newborn baby with hypotonia and ligamentous laxity having some skeletal, cardiovascular and ocular manifestations suggest about Marfan's syndrome. This is an autosomal dominant disorder with an incidence of about 1 in 10000 live births. About 15 to 30 per cent of affected individuals are due to sporadic incidence and appear as the first case in their families.

Neonatal or infantile or congenital Marfan's syndrome is a separate entity, more severe than that observed in older children. The baby presents with lax skin, hypotonia, joint laxity and dislocations, flexion contractures and arachnodactyly. The face appears to be long with large ears. The eye shows megalocornea with or without lens dislocation. Mitral regurgitation with aortic root dilation are often found on examination of the heart.

The pathogenic process is an abnormal biosynthesis of fibrillin due to a defect of 15q 21 chromosome.[2] Fibrillin is a glycoprotein constituting microfibrils which provide the scaffolding network of elastin. Many mutations of the fibrillin gene have been described.

Diagnosis

Clinical features with echocardiography help in the diagnosis. In families with affection of several members molecular genetic study helps.

Treatment

Genetic counselling is necessary because of heritable nature of the disease with many sporadic incidence. The paternal age is somewhat higher in sporadic cases than in general population among the fathers of normal babies. These are the cases representing new dominant mutations with lesser risk to the future offspring of the normal parents. The 15q 21 is inherited by each child of an affected individual causing transmission of the disease. Hence is the need for genetic counselling.

The treatment of cardiac and ocular complications will be by cardiothoracic specialist and ophthalmologist. Muscular tone is improved by regular physiotherapy. However, excessive exercise is avoided because of precipitation of cardiovascular symptoms.

WALKER-WARBURG SYNDROME

This syndrome includes hydrocephalus, agyria (lack of convolutions in the cerebral cortex) and other malformations of the brain accompanied with retinal dysplasia and encephalocele, when it is known as HARD + E. The syndrome is designated as COMS when hydrocephalus and cerebral or cerebellar malformations are associated with ocular problems and muscular dystrophy. The muscular abnormality is often hypotonia with elevation of creative kinase and myopathic changes on electromyography. This is an autosomal recessive disorder and is often lethal.

MECKEL SYNDROME

The orthopaedic problem in this syndrome is postaxial polydactyly. Other features in this lethal autosomal disorder are occipital encephalocele, hydrocephalus, cleft lip and palate, microphthalmia, fibrosis of the liver and dysplasia of the kidneys.

ELLIS-VAN CREVELD SYNDROME

Ellis-van Creveld syndrome is described with general abnormalities of skeletal development, evident at birth.

VELO-CARDIO-FACIAL SYNDROME

A newborn baby with slender and tapering fingers along with prominent and tubular nose should be looked for cleft plate and heart defects and if they occur together should be designated as velo-cardio-facial syndrome. Neonatal hypocalcaemia, which is a rare biochemical finding may occur in 13 per cent of patients. Microcephaly and ocular problems may occur.

SMITH-LEMLI-PITZ SYNDROME

In this autosomal recessive disorder intrauterine growth retardation is associated with microcephaly, celft palate, ambiguous genitalia, hypoplastic thumbs, soft tissue syndactyly of the second and third toes, postaxial polydactyly, pyloric stenosis and cardiac defects. The facial appearance is characteristic with small chin, continuity of the forehead with the nose, the normal angle at the nasal bridge being absent.

WIDERVANCK OR CERVICO-OCULO-ACOUSTIC SYNDROME

This syndrome, occurring usually in females, is an association of cleft palate with a triad of Klippel-Feil syndrome, Duane anomaly of abducens muscle palsy with retractio bulbi and nerve deafness. Sometimes renal anomalies are present.

ORAL-FACIAL-DIGITAL SYNDROME

In this syndrome of oral, facial and digital abnormality type I variety is of x-lined dominant trait, seen only in females and includes cleft lip and palate, bifid tongue with brachydactyly, syndactyly and polydactyly, involving mainly the hallux. The type II variety of the same oral, facial and digital involvement is of autosomal recessive variety and is known as Mohr syndrome.

GOLDENHAR SYNDROME

This syndrome includes hemifacial microsomia due to first and second branchial arch defect, microtia with preauricular tags, epibulbar dermoids, hypoplasia of mandibular ramus and condyle, vertebral defects in little less than half of the cases and in some cardiac and renal defects.

TREACHER COLLINS SYNDROME (MANDIBULO-FACIAL DYSOSTOSIS)

This is a bilaterally symmetric autosomal dominant disorder of face with malar hypoplasia, down-slanting palpebral fissures, lower lid colobomas with absence of lower lashes, external ear defects and mandibular hypoplasia. Cleft palate is frequently associated and rarely congenital heart disease. When limb anomaly in the form of (post axial) (ulnar ray) limb defect is associated the condition is known as Miller syndrome and when preaxial (radial ray) limb defect is found it is known as Nager acrofacial dysostosis. The Miller syndrome is autosomal recessive in inheritance and the last one is due to both autosomal recessive and dominant inheritance.

MÖBIUS SYNDROME

This syndrome includes hypodactyly specially of the hands with hypoglossia and VI and VII cranial nerve deficiency. Glossopalatine ankylosis is a rare association.

EEC OR EARLY AMNION DISRUPTION SYNDROME

Early rupture of amnion is not too infrequent a defect, usually asymmetric, may cause haemorrhage and necrosis of a previously normal limb. The residual bands of amnion may lead to congenital amputations or deep circumferential constriction rings. The features are described in detail in a separate chapter.

SCALP DEFECT—ECTRODACTYLY SYNDROME OR ADAMS-OLIVER SYNDROME

This syndrome includes cutaneous aplasia over bone defect in the skull with minimal digital hypoplasia to asymmetric transverse terminal defects of the hands and feet. In this autosomal dominant inheritance there may be variants like aplasia cutis at different sites.

CORNELIA DE LANGE'S OR BRACHMANN DE LANGE SYNDROME

In this syndrome there is characteristic facies with down-turned upper lip and a long prominent philtrum with prenatal growth deficiency and mental retardation. The baby is hirshute with hypoplastic short limbs.

THROMBOCYTOPENIA-ABSENT RADIUS SYNDROME

Here hypoplasia of the thumbs is associated with defects of the radius. Thrombocytopenia is transiently present in these babies only in infancy. The inheritance is of autosomal recessive type and there is frequent occurrence of other skeletal anomalies with infrequent cardiac abnormality.

ASPHYXIATING THORACIC DYSTROPHY (JEUNE SYNDROME)

In this syndrome the ribs are broad and short and the thorax is rigid. Some degree of lung hypoplasia may also be present. The severely affected babies suffer from respiratory distress from birth. The kidneys may show cystic hypoplasia resulting in hypertension and renal failure. This syndrome is part of a generalised chondrodystrophy. There is metaphyseal irregularity with short extremities and postaxial polydactyly. The inheritance is of autosomal recessive type.

RUBINSTEIN-TAYBI SYNDROME

In this syndrome of sporadic occurrence the suffering babies will have broad thumbs and big toes with a facies presenting down-slanting palpebral fissures, beaked nose having cataract with colobomas of the iris in the eyes and hypoplasia of the maxilla.

BECKWITH-WIEDEMANN SYNDROME

This syndrome is often presented with hemihypertrophy of one side of the body which may be larger in circumference and/or length. The contralateral side of the body has a chance of developing an embryonal tumour like Wilms' tumour, adrenal cortical carcinoma, hepatoblastoma and others. Macroglossia, omphalocele and posterior ear pits are characteristic findings. Hypoglycaemia and polycythaemia may be detected in the neonatal period. Duplication of 11p15 as a chromosome anomaly is detected in many patients.

REFERENCES

1. Nelson Textbook of Pediatrics; 16th edn, 2 Vols; ed by R.E. Berhman, RM Kliegman, HB Jenson. Singapore, Harcourt Asia: WB Saunders Co; 2000 (printed in India).p.327.
2. Robinson LK in Nelson Textbook Pediatrics; 16th edn 2131.

Chapter 39

Neonatal Gangrene

Keywords: Gangrene in a neonate is very rare in occurrence-babies of diabetic mothers have been reported to suffer from-culture from areas of necrosis repeatedly prove to be sterile on many occasions-the use of prophylactic γ-globulin and infusion of donor neutrophils-fascinating and Jones soft compression dressing are of help.

NEONATAL GANGRENE

Gangrene in a neonate mostly involving the lower extremities is very rare in occurrence. About sixty cases.[1,2] have been reported in the literature of which half the cases had the manifestation of gangrene on the first day of life. Embolic manifestation due to thrombi originating in the umbilical veins[3] or arteries[4] or in terminal aorta or iliac vessels or in renal or adrenal veins[5] has been attributed as the cause leading to ischaemia and decreased perfusion. In the case of gangrene occurring in the upper extremity no definite cause of thrombi has been found except in one case where the thrombus was reported to occur in the vessels arising from the aortic arch.[3] Neonatal gangrene has been reported to occur among three babies delivered by diabetic mothers with long history of diabetes.[1]

Predisposing Conditions

Some predisposing conditions leading to development of thrombi with their embolic manifestation have been described in the literature. Umbilical artery catheterisation, venepuncture or a cutdown, disseminated intravascular coagulations, wrapping the extremity too tightly are the predisposing causes. Association of congenital heart disease, sepsis, dehydration, polycythaemia has been found in some cases. Uterine trauma associated with placental bands, encircling umbilical cords, amniotic bands encircling a toe or a finger, prolapse of the affected limb between the uterine wall and the presenting head, spontaneous rupture of membranes and difficult delayed labour are all attributed as the cause.

In the three babies of diabetic mother the suggestive cause was localised thrombosis of small veins in the arms. There was an incidence of 15.8 per cent of venous thrombosis in babies of diabetic mothers which was 0.8 per cent in babies of nondiabetic mothers.[6]

Local and Systemic Examination

On local examination the baby may show a markedly edematous area of the affected part with occasional blisters and cyanosis of proximal areas. The edema increases and the affected limb shows some tightness due to accumulation of edema fluids. The capillary filling decreases in the distal area and the radial or posterior tibial pulse become nonpalpable according to the area of affection. Spontaneous movements of digits could rarely be seen. Systemically, the babies may show evidence of congenital heart disease or a list of other causes mentioned before. The babies of diabetic mother may have excessive birth weight, enlarged umbilical cord, hepatomegaly and cardiomyopathy. The radiographic features of the affected part may be normal.

Treatment

The treatment of the condition is fasciotomy of the affected part after preoperative application of antibiotic preferably on the first day of life. Muscle tissues are often found necrotic without any signs of contraction on stimulation. Providone-iodine and fine mesh dressing with a Jones soft compression dressing on most occasions help in the return of the capillary refilling and the pulse. Multiple dressings are necessary and antibiotics after culture are continued. The use of prophylactic g-globulin and infusion of donor neutrophils have been reported. Cultures from areas of necrosis repeatedly prove to be sterile on many occasions. Split skin grafting is necessary to cover area of affection as the condition of the wound permits. Although the circulation improves, the condition leaves behind some residual motor power weakness.

REFERENCES

1. Hensinger RN. Gangrene of the newborn—A case report. J Bone Joint Sug 1975;57A:121.
2. Hensinger RN, Jones ET. Neonatal orthopedics. New York: Grune and Stratton; 1981.pp.88-9.
3. Braly BD. Neonatal arterial thrombosis and embolism. Surgery 1965;58: 869.
4. Gross RE. Arterial embolism and thrombosis in infancy. Am J Dis child 1945;70: 61.
5. Valderrama E, Gribetz I, Strauss L. Peripheral gangrene in a newborn infant associated with renal and adrenal vein thrombosis. J Pediatr 1972;80:101.
6. Oppenheimer EH, Esterly JR. Thrombosis in the newborn: Comparison between infants of diabetic and nondiabetic mothers. J Pediatric 1965;67:549.

Chapter 40

Rheumatic Disorders Manifesting in the Neonatal Period

Keywords: Systemic lupus erythematosus (SLE) and antiphospholipid antibody syndrome without arthritis manifest in neonates–outcome depends upon the presence of antiphospholipid antibiotics, anti Ro/SS-A and anti La/SS-B auto-antibiotics.

SYSTEMIC LUPUS ERYTHEMATOSUS

Systemic lupus erythematosus (SLE) and antiphospholipid antibody syndrome manifest in neonates with their characteristic symptoms. But, fortunately, none of them present with arthritis.

Systemic lupus erythematosus is often diagnosed in women of childbearing age. If the disease is controlled during the second and third trimester of pregnancy the outcome is better. Association of sicca syndrome in about 30 per cent cases of SLE is due to the presence of La (SS-B) and Ro (SS-A) antigen. Antiphospholipid syndrome with its arterial and venous occlusive features, cutaneous, renal and cardiac manifestations may be associated with SLE.

Neonatal outcome depends upon the presence of antiphospholipid antibodies, anti Ro/SS-A and anti La/SS-B auto-antibodies. Toxic immunosuppressive medications during pregnancy also influence the outcome. When the risk for positive auto-antibodies of SLE in a newborn is about 10 percent, the risk for clinical manifestation of SLE is only 1 percent.

Neonatal lupus erythematosus syndrome manifests with features of skin rash, thrombocytopenia, liver function defects, congenital heart block but seldom arthritis. To avert congenital heart block, the incidence of which is fortunately very rare, foetal monitoring for bradycardia and echocardiography during 20 and 24 weeks of gestation is mandatory. The treatment of SLE during pregnancy is done with usual antirheumatic drugs and steroid, avoiding toxic immunosuppressive agents like azathioprine, cyclophosphamide, methotrexate, etc.

Chapter 41

Neonatal Malignancy and Sacrococcygeal Teratoma

Keywords: Neonatal malignant tumour is rare–embryonic rhabdomyosacroma, a malignant tumour in a seven days old infant has been reported–sacrococcygeal Teratoma may occur in the newborn–benign in nature.

NEONATAL MALIGNANCY

Although bone tumours are not common in the early pediatric age group, Wilms' tumour and tumours around the eye and orbit like retinoblastoma, metastatic neuroblastoma and cancer are found in early infancy. An embryonic rhabdomyosarcoma in a seven days old neonate has been reported by Desai.[1]

No particular maternal factor can be mentioned as the supporting cause in the mesodermal tumors in the neonates. Environmental factors have got no role in neonatal cancers. No genetic cause can be attributed and immunodeficiency at such an earlier age can rarely be thought about.

The clinical finding of an abdominal lump of renal origin suggesting a Wilms' tumour in a neonate has not been observed by the author. But the presence of such a lump with congenital abnormalities like hemihypertrophy and aniridia arouse a strong suspicion of the diagnosis of Wilms' tumour. A similar tumour, a neuroblastoma arising from the neural crest is found in the same situation as above and mimic a Wilms' tumour. The incidence of neuroblastoma in neonates has not been found in the literature. The tumour may present in different stages of maturation. The neuroblastoma is the most malignant, but the other two differentiated ones like ganglioneuroblastoma and ganglioneuroma are comparatively benign in nature. A large percentage of these tumours secrete catecholamines, which is of great diagnostic importance.

Renal angiographic studies and inferior venacavagram helps in the diagnosis of Wilms' tumour. Bone marrow study to show pseudorosette formation, X-rays to show soft tissue shadow of abdominal mass and metastasis to skull, orbit and spine, inferior venacavagram and increased secretion of catecholamines help in the diagnosis of neuroblastoma.

Rhabdomyosarcoma is a common form of malignant lesion in early infancy. The embryonic form is the most common one in an infant. The lesion, common in various soft tissues, the urogenital tract, the orbit and the nasopharynx starts to grow rapidly from nodular lesion and metastasise early to the lymph nodes and then to the lungs, mediastinum, liver and skeleton.

The treatment of these tumours in general is surgical excision followed by radiotherapy and chemotherapy. Rhabdomyosarcoma which was once thought as radioresistant has been found to be responding well to radiotherapy and chemotherapy.

Although occurrence of rhabdomyosarcoma in a neonate has been reported, neonatal incidence of bone tumour has not been found yet in the literature.

SACROCOCCYGEAL TERATOMA

These neoplasms contain derivatives of more than one of the three primary germinal layers of the embryo and present mostly in the sacrococcygeal area in the newborn and hence called sacrococcygeal teratomas. These teratomas are solid tumours, usually present in the newborn and are mostly benign. Females are twice or even four times more affected than the males. The detection of the tumour may happen in the prenatal period or after birth. Congenital anomalies like genitourinary, hind gut and lower vertebral malformations are often associated with this condition.

The tumour occurs in association with polyhydramnios and dystocia and may present in four different types. The type I is predominantly external, having minimum presacral component, with an incidence of 46.6 per cent of all sacrococcygeal teratomas, with no metastasis and hence a mortality rate of 11 per cent, the lowest among all types. The benign nature depends upon the presence of mature tissues and not embryonic tissues. The type II has lesser external presentation than type I with quite a big pelvic extension. The incidence is 34.6 per cent, metastatic rate 6 per cent and a little higher mortality rate of 18 per cent than the previous type. The type III is predominantly internal with a huge abdominopelvic mass and having small external presentation. The incidence is 8.8 per cent, with highest metastatic rate of all varieties of 20 per cent and considerable mortality of 28 per cent. The last and the type IV is presented purely presacrally without any external presentation having a frequency of 10 per cent, the metastatic rate of 8 per cent but quite a high mortality rate of 21 per cent. The teratomas may occur in other locations also but usually in the midline in the childhood variety. The type of teratoma occurring at puberty mostly occur from the ovary.

The diagnosis is made usually from the external appearance and occasionally from a routine rectal examination. The functional problems with bladder, bowel, lymphatic channels and blood vessels are not too many even with a large benign tumour. The problem of painful defection is quite common. Major functional problems indicate towards malignant nature of the condition.

The condition is to be differentiated from meningomyelocoeles, from pelvic neuroblastomas in highly undifferentiated type and in smaller sized varieties from pilonidal cysts. The variety with painful defection is to be differentiated from rectal abscess.

Early surgical excision with excision of the entire coccyx, to which the tumour is attached, is the hallmark of treatment. Failure to do early surgery will lead to proliferation of undifferentiated variety, when present, and hence a bad prognosis.

REFERENCE

1. Desai PB. Malignant disease in childhood. In Udani PM (Ed): Textbook of Pediatrics 3: 2426-45.

Chapter 42

Conjoined (Siamese) Twins

Keywords: Conjoined twins—ischiopagus—musculoskeletal problems in separation.

CONJOINED (SIAMESE) TWINS

Twin babies, joined together through some connections lead to a separate entity of conjoined twins or Siamese twins with an incidence of 1 in 50,000. The site of connections varies and the names of the conjoined twins are according to the connections. The highest incidence is of thoraco-omphalopagus, 28 percent of all conjoined twins; thoracopagus (18%), omphalopagus (10%), craniopagus (6%), incomplete duplication (10%).[1] The possible cause of development of conjoined twins is relatively late monovular separation. Many of the conjoined twins are females. The surgical separation becomes difficult with the degree of sharing of vital organs.

The author was the chief of the orthopaedic team during separation of ischiopagus tetrapus twins (Fig. 42.1) and observed the musculoskeletal problems during the separation.[2] The successful separation we performed was a staged procedure. The gastrointestinal tracts were separated at a preliminary operation[3] and the definitive operation was performed three months later. Skeletal reconstruction was performed concurrently during the separation, the earlier of its kind and the only one was from Kualalumpur.[4] Staging

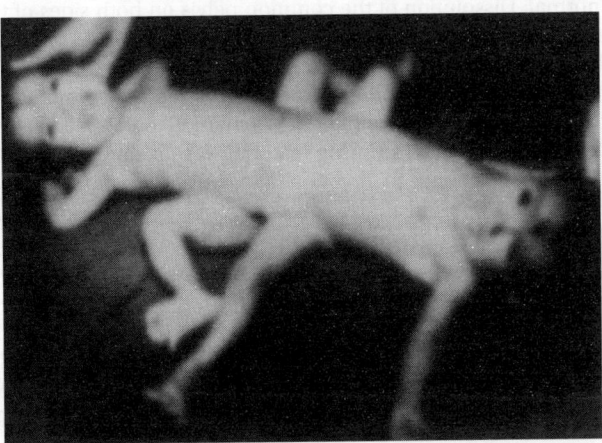

Fig. 42.1: Ischiopagus tetrapus conjoined twins

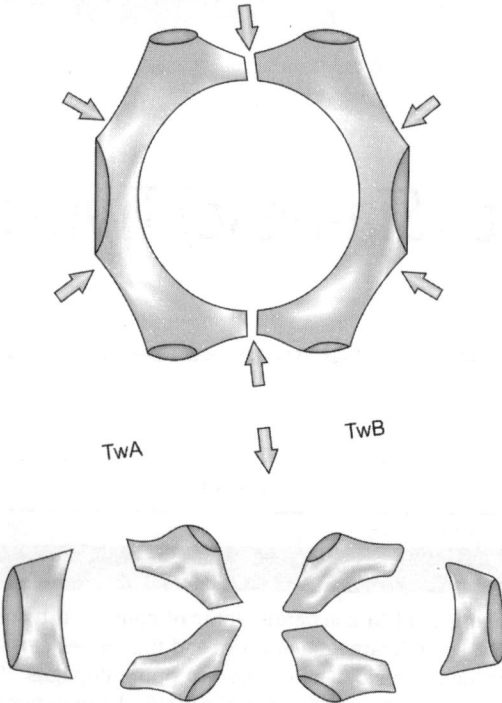

Fig. 42.2: Complex 'O' shaped common pelvis in conjoined twins before and after separation

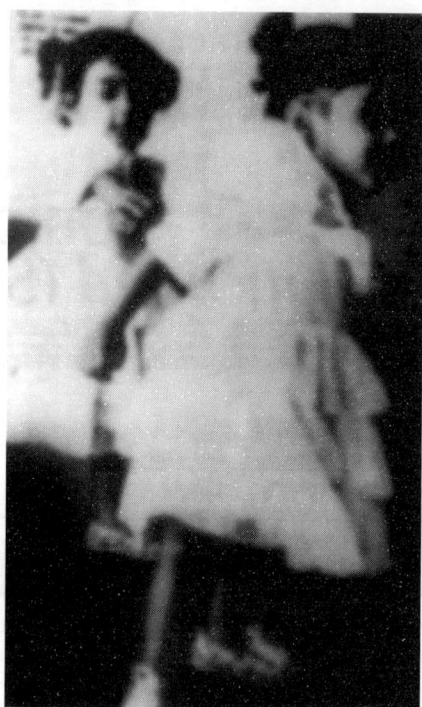

Fig. 42.3: The two babies one and a half years after separation

permitted performance of the final separation on healthier babies with exclusion of the intestinal contents from the wounds and with a reduced operating time. During skeletal separation we had the problem of a complex 'O' shaped common pelvis with two sacrums facing each other (Fig. 42.2) the pubis of one twin of one side joining with the pubis of the opposite side of the other twin, with the femora at right angles at the hips, which were normal. Dissolution of the common pelvis on both sides of the sacrums with wide separation of the iliac fragments by iliac osteotomies accomplished closure of the widely separated pubes of the respective twins. Subperiosteal erasing of the gluteal muscles from the iliums helped in obtaining wide separation of the iliac fragments. The curved incisions for four iliac osteotomies, which were deviations from the usual vertical incisions, helped in maintaining circulation to the skin flaps.

To prevent sinus formation 'O' Vicryl suturing material was used for apposition of the pubic bones. After the pubes were sutured, the change in direction of the lower part of the psoas muscles from a near-horizontal to a near-vertical position must have caused tightness in the psoas, leading to postoperative flexion contracture in the hips, which became normal later on with skin traction. On the other hand, the change in the direction of the rectus abdominis and pubococcygeus after reconstruction helped to strengthen the anterior abdominal wall and the pelvic floor, respectively.

The conjoined female twins were born on November 12, 1985 and the intestinal separation was performed on August 9, 1986. The final separation was performed three months later, on November 15, 1986. Fig. 42.3 shows the two babies one and a half years after separation. The 15-year-old girls can now run, having no problems regarding locomotion, but have had recurrent urinary problems.

REFERENCES

1. Nelson. Textbook of Pediatrics 16th edn, 2 Vols. E Behrman, Robert M Kliegman, Hal B Jenson (Eds) Singapore: WB Saunders Co; 2000.p.475.
2. De Mazumder N, Chatterjee SK, Chakraborty T, Chakraborty A, Deb Maulik T, Sen MK. Musculoskeletal Problems in the separation of ischiopagus tetrapus twins (case report). J Ped Orthop 1991;11:386-91.
3. Chatterjee SK, Chakraborty AK, Deb Maulik TK, De Mazumder N, Sen MK. Staging the separation of ischiopagus twins. J Pediatr Surg 1988;23:73-5.
4. Somasundaram K, Wong KS. Ischiopagus tetrapus conjoined twins. Br J Surg 1986;73:738-41.

Chapter 43

Caffey's Disease

Keywords: Caffey and Silverman first described – fever and hyperirritability in a newborn baby with periosteal and soft tissues swelling with high ESR – no infective cause detected – self-limiting.

CAFFEY'S DISEASE

This self-limiting disease characterised by swelling of the soft tissues and the underlying bony cortex and periosteum with fever and hyperirritability usually manifests between birth and five months of age of the baby. Caffey and Silverman[1] first described this entity in detail in 1945 and hence the name.

Etiology

The cause is unknown. From the clinical behaviour, infection, either viral or bacterial, has been suggested as the cause. But no causative organism has been isolated. Hereditary factor is a possible suggestion along with allergic factor, because the disease often responds to corticosteroids.

Pathology

Inflammatory in nature the disease affects the periosteum and the surrounding soft tissues with subperiosteal bone formation resulting in cortical thickening. The swelling is associated with high leucocyte count and raised ESR. Alkaline phosphatase is also raised. The resolution is automatic with reversion to normalcy.

Clinical Features

The baby presents usually with swelling over the mandible and forearm, where ulna is affected. Mandible is the most common site of affection. Other bones are also involved like clavicle, scapula and other long bones and sometimes the disease manifests with bilateral affection. The onset is acute. The affected areas are swollen and painful. The baby is hyperirritable, sometimes associated with fever. As has been mentioned there is very high leucocyte count of about 20 to 25 thousand with high polymorphs. The ESR is raised. Culture and biopsy never proved any definite organism or infection. The swellings have remissions and exacerbations and normally subside in four to six weeks time, leaving no residual defect on most occasions.

Diagnosis

The disease affecting infants within five months of age with inflammatory swelling over the mandible, clavicle, scapula and long bones associated with slight fever and hyperirritability, raised leucocyte count and ESR is a strong suspicion of Caffey's disease. The characteristic radiographic features of diaphyseal bone formation with periosteal reaction, which follow soft tissue swelling make the suspicion even more strong.

The condition is differentiated from ost eomyelitis, Ewing's tumor, metastasis from neuroblastoma, trauma, syphilis, hypervitaminosis A. The self limiting character of the disease with subsidence of all the clinical and radiological features within a very short time make the condition different from other conditions mentioned above.

Treatment

No definite treatment is necessary. Rest and analgesics and only rarely corticosteroids are necessary to minimise the swelling.

REFERENCE

1. Caffey J, Silverman WA. Infantile cortical hyperostosis - preliminary report in a new syndrome. AJR 1945;54:1.

Chapter 44

Syndromes having Craniosynostosis Presenting at Birth

Keywords: Craniosynostosis with craniofacial defects - apert, Crouzon, Pfeiffer, Saethre-chotzen, Antley-Bixler are only few of about fifty syndromes - all are with limb and/or vertebral defects.

CRANIOSYNOSTOSIS

Craniosynostosis occurs due to premature fusion of one or more cranial sutures. The head size is deformed as a result of the fusion. The deformity may occur alone or in association with other malformations. The incidence is 1 in 2500 live births.[1] Genetic inheritance is found in almost all cases.

According to the fusion of a particular suture the shape of the head changes. Bilateral coronal suture fusion leads to brachycephaly—usually a short and wide cranium, occasionally may be tall; unilateral coronal suture fusion results in a plagiocephaly, i.e. flattening of one half of the forehead with flattening of occiput on the contralateral side. These two deformities produce 25 per cent of cases and mostly affect females. Eight percent of cases are familial.

Other varieties are scaphocephaly with long narrow cranium having prominent forehead and occiput; trigonocephaly with pointed and prominant forehead is due to premature fusion of metopic suture. A severe form, known as Kleeblattschadel[2] is a cloverleaf shaped head due to premature fusion of multiple sutures. About 40 per cent of this deformity is found in thanatophoric dysplasia and 20 per cent in Pfeiffer syndrome. The most common craniosynostosis of about 50 per cent incidence is due to simple unilateral sagittal suture synostosis. Two percent of cases are familial.

Of about fifty syndromes in which craniosynostosis occurs only the most common ones and those with orthopaedic problems will be described below. Mental retardation is a common feature in all the varieties. Neurological evaluation is done in all cases. Early surgery helps in improving the contour of the cranium helping in better growth of the brain.

Apert Syndrome

This inherited deformity is of autosomal dominant type.[3] The characteristics of craniofacial defects are tall brachycephalic skull due to bilateral coronal sutural synostosis with hydrocephalus and large anterior fontanel, hypoplastic midface with beaked nose, cleft but high arched narrow palate and deafness of conductive type.

The limb problems are of cutaneous and bony syndactyly between second, third and fourth digits of hands and feet. The syndrome has had other features of cardiovascular defects with infrequent occurrence of tracheo-esophageal fistula, esophageal atresia and pyloric stenosis.

Crouzon Syndrome

The characteristic malformations of this autosomal dominant syndrome are cervical vertebral fusion and stiff elbows with craniofacial defects. Here again the coronal sutural synostosis leads to brachycephaly with midface hypoplasia, prognathism, high arched but narrow palate, shallow orbits with proptosis and like Apert syndrome conductive deafness.

Pfeiffer Syndrome

The tall brachycephalic skull is known as Kleeblattschädel looks like cloverleaf having a bad prognosis even with surgery, associated with hydrocephalus, ocular hypertelorism with downslanting palpebral fissure. The nose is beaked and the palate is high arched.

The limb defects are limited to broad thumbs and great toes. Pyloric stenosis and malpositioned anus are not very frequent in occurrence.

The inheritance is of autosomal dominant type.

Other Brachycephalic Synostosis

Saethre - Chotzen syndrome and Antley-Bixler syndrome, both show ear and hand problems besides brachycephaly, but the former is autosomal dominant in inheritance and the latter of autosomal recessive type.

Saethre - Chotzen syndrome shows brachy and plagiocephaly with low frontal hairline, ptosis and prominent crus of the ears. With cutaneous syndactyly occasionally congenital problems of heart, kidney and testes are found.

Antley-Bixler syndrome shows a trapezoid shaped head, depressed nasal bridge, choanal atresia and dysplastic ears. In the upper limbs, radiohumeral synostosis and joint contractures are associated with arachnodactyly. Like the former variety congenital heart and renal problems of infrequent occurrence are associated with imperforate anus, genital and vertebral anomalies.

Other Varieties

The extreme variety of Kleeblattschädel with depressed nasal bridge and retrogressed midface is found in thanatophoric dysplasia. The stature is short with very short limbs and narrow thorax. This is a sporadic variety and is lethal in the neonatal period.

Other craniosynostosis are associated with cutaneous syndactyly and broad thumbs. One of the two varieties as described by Greig is presented with infrequent scaphocephaly, frontal bossing, hypertelorism, pre and post-axial polydactyly.

The other variety is of craniofrontonasal dysplasia having coronal synostosis with hypertelorism and bifid nasal tip. Besides cutaneous syndactyly and broad thumbs the nails are grooved and the shoulders are sloping in association with scoliosis.

REFERENCES

1. Hunter AGW, Rudd NL. Craniosynostosis I. Sagittal synostosis: Its genetics and associated clinical findings in 214 patients who lacked involvement of the coronal suture(s). Teratology 1976;14:185-93.
2. William Taeusch, Robefita. A Ballard, Mary Ellen Avery (Eds). Schaffer and Avery's Diseases of the Newborn, 6th edn. Philadelphia, London: WB Saunders Co, Harcourt Brace Jovanovich, Inc 172.
3. Cohen MM Jr. Craniosynostosis update 1987. Am J Med Genet 1988;4:99-148.

Chapter 45

Chondrodysplasia Punctata

Keywords: Two varieties of chondrodysplasia–epiphyeal stippling–short long bones–joint contractures–vertebral anomalies–severe rhizomelic type is autosomal recessive–Conradi-Hunermann type may be autosomal dominant in some and recessive in others.

SEVERE RHIZOMELIC TYPE

The condition manifests at birth affecting equally in both sexes with very short limbs, flat face, depressed bridge of nose, frequent occurrence of bilateral cataract with occasional presence of a variety of skin disorders and vertebral anomalies.[1] Congenital heart disease, tracheo-oesophageal fistula, imperforate anus may occasionally be associated. The baby suffers from mental retardation and optic atrophy. The joints show contractures and the hip is congenitally dislocated.

Radiographically stippling of the epiphysis is a characteristic sign with extra-cartilaginous calcification. Dwarfism is present in the long bones which are extremely short with metaphyseal cupping and splaying. Separate centers of ossification for the vertebral bodies, one for the anterior part and one for the posterior part of the body may be present. Vertebral anomalies result into scoliosis.

This is a condition of autosomal recessive inheritance. Parental consanguinity has been reported with kindreds having affected sibs.

Pathologically, there is gross abnormality of the enchondral bone formation with reduced vascularity and little calcification. Polymorphous chalky deposits of circumscribed nature is the cause of stippling found radiographically.[2]

The condition will have to be differentiated from multiple epiphyseal dysplasia with multiple epiphyseal ossification centers which mimic stippling but are easily identified because of their larger sizes.[3] Prenatal infections, sometimes found in chromosomal anomalies and in cerebrohepatorenal syndrome may show congenital stippling of epiphyses; vertebral epiphyses being free from stippling.

The prognosis is bad and babies suffering from this disease die of respiratory infection and seldom cross the first year of life.

CONRADI-HUNERMANN TYPE

This is a mild variety of the previous type and many of the features are common. There is confusion about the genetic inheritance—some of autosomal dominant, some of recessive inheritance. Sporadic cases are also reported.

Females are two or three times more affected than males. The milder forms may not be recognized at birth. Contractures of different joints like shoulder, hip and knee with shortening of only one limb are chracteristics of this condition. Proximal limb bones are short. Other clinical and radiological features are almost same as the first type but of lesser magnitude.

Pathologically, endochondral bone formation is not affected at all unlike the first type but the epiphyseal cartilage shows cysts and also calcification.

Differential diagnosis will be as described in the first type.

Some of the children with the above features may be still born or die in the perinatal period. If they survive the life expectancy is normal and epiphyseal stippling disappear by about four years of age but later develop epiphyseal changes in those areas.

Surviving children will require limb lengthening of the affected short limb and correction of scoliosis. Skin condition which may not be as worse as the first type may require treatment occasionally.

REFERENCES

1. Wynne-Davis R, Fairbank TJ. Fairbank's Atlas of General Affections of the Skeleton, 2nd edn. Edinburgh: Churchill Livingstone; 1976.p.10.
2. Selakovich WG, Warren White J. Chondrodystrophia calcificans congenita. J Bone and Joint Surg 1955;37A:1271.
3. Silverman FN. Discussion on the relation between stippled epiphyses and the multiplex form of epiphyseal dysplasia. Birth Defects original Article Series 5, Part 4, 68; quoted by Wynne-Davies R. and Fairbank TJ in their Atlas, 10.

Index

Page numbers followed by *f* refer to figure

A
Abdomen 7
Abnormal maturation of growth-plate condroblasts 21
Abnormality of genes causing genetic disorders 13
Acetabular index 105*f*
Achler's Dunlop syndrome 93
Achondrogenesis 14, 20, 21, 24
Achondroplasia 17, 20-22, 23*f*
Acrocephalosyndactyly 20, 21, 32
Acute
    osteomyelitis 142
    psoas abscess 148
Adams-Oliver syndrome 156
Aitken's classification 63*f*
Alpha foetoprotein 18
Amputation 47
Amyoplasia 88
Anatomy of radial club hand 131
Antitetanus serum 152
Apert syndrome 20, 21, 32, 168
Apgar score 11
Arthrogryposis
    like deformities 89
    multiplex congenita 88, 90*f*, 96*f*
Asphyxiating thoracic dysplasia 20, 21, 32, 156
Atresia choanae 17
Australia antigen 17
Autosomal
    dominant inheritance 14
    recessive inheritance 14

B
Beckwith-Wiedemann syndrome 156
Bent bones in
    neonate 51
    osteogenesis imperfecta 30*f*
Bilateral
    club foot deformities 81*f*
    congenital subluxation of knees 97*f*
    dislocation of hips 90*f*
Birth
    fractures 39
    injuries 38
    of brachial plexus 41
    weight 11
Bone
    dysplasias 20, 21
    injuries 38
Brachial plexus injuries 38
Brachmann De Lange syndrome 156
Brachycephalic synostosis 169

C
Caffey's disease 166
Campomelic dysplasia 20
Camptodactyly 139
Caput succedaneum 39
Care
    and feeding of premature infants 2
    of newborn 1
Carpenter's syndrome 20, 138
Cartilaginous dysplasias 20, 21
Cause of genetic disorders 15
Central core disease 33, 34
Cephalhaematoma 38
Cerebral palsy 36
Cervical spine injury 40
Chondrodysplasia punctata 14, 19-21, 170
Chondroectodermal dysplasia 20, 21, 31
Chromosomes 13
Classification of limb deficiencies 46
Cleft foot deformity 76
Cleidocranial
    dysostosis 127
    dysplasia 14, 20
Clinodactyly 139
Closed spina bifida 114
Clostridium tetani 152
Club foot 78, 83, 85
    deformity 96*f*
Coarctation of aorta 134
Coloboma 17
Communicating hydrocephalus 134
Complete paraxial hemimelia of fibula 46*f*
Complex deformity of kyphoscoliosis 51
Congenital
    abduction contracture of hip and pelvic obliquity 111
    absence of pectoral muscles 127, 128
    anomalies 16
    clasped thumb 139
    constriction
        band syndrome 47
        ring completely encircling left leg 48*f*
    convex pes valgus 74
    coxa vara 66
    defects of femur 56
    developmental anomalies of extremities in neonate 44
    dislocation of
        hip 100, 102
        knee 96*f*
        patella 98
    hallux varus 76
    high scapula 123
    kyphoscoliosis tibia and fibula 51, 52*f*
    laxity of joints 93
    longitudinal deficiency of fibula 59, 60f, 61*f*
    thumb 138
    tibia 57, 58f, 134
    ulna 131
    lower limb defects 56
    malformations 12, 16
    metatarsus varus 73
    muscular
        dystrophy 33
        torticollis 121
    myotonic dystrophy 33, 35
    pseudoarthrosis of
        clavicle 125
        fibula 54, 55
        tibia 54, 54*f*
    radioulnar synostosis 129, 130*f*
    scoliosis 114, 117, 117*f*
    short femur 56, 57
    structural myopathies 33, 34
    subluxation
        and dislocations around knee 96
        of left knee 97*f*

synostosis of elbow 129, 130
talipes calcaneovalgus 74
trigger thumb 140
Conjoined twins 163
Conradi disease 19-21
Cornelia De Lange
    syndrome 21, 32, 138, 156
Craig splint 107f
Craniocarpotarsal syndrome 21
Craniosynostosis 168
Creatine phosphokinase 33
Crouzon syndrome 169
Cytomegalovirus 17

D
Denis-Browne splint 84
Deoxyribonucleic acid 13
Depressed fracture 40
Detection of musculoskeletal
    abnormalities in neonatal period 9
Development of vertebral bodies 113
Developmental dysplasia of hip 100
Diagnosis of developmental
    dysplasia of hip 102
Diaphyseal
    aclasis 20
    dysplasia 20
Diastrophic
    dwarfism 14
    dysplasia 21, 24
Disorders of voluntary muscles 33
Distal arthrogryposis 93
Down syndrome 17, 18, 94, 139, 153
Dyschondroplasia 20
Dysplasia 16
    of hip 100

E
Early amnion disruption
    syndrome 156
Ectrodactyly syndrome 156
Electromyography 33
Ellis-Van Creveld
    syndrome 20, 21, 31, 155
Enchondromatosis 20
Equinovalgus foot 60f
Equinovarus deformity 90f
Erb's palsy 40
Escobar syndrome 21
Etiology of club foot 79
Excision of kyphotic vertebrae 115

F
Face 7
Fairbank's triangle 67f
Fanconi
    anaemia 21
syndrome 138
Femoral hypoplasia 56
Fetal alcohol syndrome 93
Flexion deformities of fingers 136f
Foetal
    alcohol syndrome 21
    dwarfism 21
    face syndrome 20, 21
Folate deficiency 17
Fracture of
    clavicle 40
    shaft of
        femur 41
        humerus 40
Freeman-Sheldon
    syndrome 21, 93
    whistling face syndrome 88

G
Genetically determined myopathy 33
Glenoidal labrum 102
Goldenhar syndrome 155
Growth and development of
    neonate 6

H
Haemophilus influenzae 143
Hallermann-Streiff syndrome 21
Hand reduction malformations 140
Head
    and neck injuries 38
    and upper limb syndrome 20, 21
    circumference 11
Heart defect 17
Hereditary
    multiple exostoses 20
    progressive arthro-
        ophthalmopathy 20
Hilgenreiner's
    epiphyseal angle 68f
    line 68f
Holt-Oram syndrome 134, 138
Horner's syndrome 42
Hurler syndrome 150
Hyperthermia 89
Hypertrophied ligamentum
    teres 102

I
Imperforate anus 134
Infantile spinal muscular
    atrophy 33, 35
Inherited neonatal orthopaedic
    conditions 14
Instability of hip 64
Intercalary
    congenital limb deficiency 45f
deficiencies 46
Intra-abdominal injuries 38
Intra-cranial haemorrhage 39
Intra-uterine
    environmental factors 89
    growth retardation 10
Ischiopagus tetrapus conjoined
    twins 163f

J
Jeune's disease 14, 20, 21, 32, 156
Joshi's external stabilization system
    fixator 92

K
Kirner deformity 139
Klippel-Feil syndrome 17, 119
Knee joint 144f
Kniest
    disease 20, 21, 24
    syndrome 14
Kyphoscoliosis 51
    of tibia and fibula 30f

L
Larsen syndrome 88, 93
Linear fracture 40
Lobster claw 76
Longitudinal deficiency of thumb 138
Lower
    arm type of Klumpke 41
    limb 7
        anomalies 51
        deformities 92
        rotation 71

M
Macrodactyly 77
Malrotation and inadequate
    proximal musculature 65
Mandibular hypoplasia 21
Mandibulofacial dysostosis 155
Marfan's syndrome 93, 154
Maternal
    infections 17
    Rh isoimmunisation 17
Meckel syndrome 154
Melnick-Needle syndrome 20
Melorheostosis 20
Mesomelic dysplasias 20, 21
Metaphyseal chondrodysplasia 21
Metatarsus
    adductus 73
    primus varus 76
Metatropic
    dwarfism 14
    dysplasia 20-22

Index

Micrognathia 16f
Mid-arm circumference 11
Miscellaneous finger deformities 139
Mitochondrial and storage myopathies 33, 34
Möbius syndrome 17, 156
Moro reflex 42
Morquio's syndrome 25
Mucolipidoses 150
Multiple pterygium syndrome 21
Myotonia congenita 33, 34

N
Nail-patella syndrome 20
Nemaline myopathy 33, 34
Neonatal
　deformities of toes 76
　gangrene 158
　infections 142
　malignancy 161
　orthopaedic 1
　　diseases 13
　osteomyelitis 142, 143f-146f
　rickets 21, 49, 50f
　tetanus 152
Nerve injuries 38
Noonan syndrome 94

O
Occipital osteodiastasis 40
Oculodento-osseous dysplasia 21
Oculomandibulofacial syndrome 21
Oesophageal atresia 134
Ollier's disease 20
Open spina bifida 114
Oral-facial-digital syndrome 21, 155
Osteochondromatosis 20
Osteodysplasty 20
Osteogenesis imperfecta 14, 20, 25, 26f, 27f, 29f, 30f
　congenita 21
Osteo-onycho dysplasia 20
Osteopetrosis congenita 20, 21, 31
Osteoporosis in osteogenesis imperfecta 31f
Osteoporotic bones 50f

P
Pancytopenia-dysmeila syndrome 21
Papillon-Leage syndrome 21
Pauwel's Y osteotomy 69f
Pavlik harness 108f
Pedunculated encephalocoele 134
Pfeiffer syndrome 169
Phocomelia in left lower limb 45f
Pierre Robin syndrome 16f, 17, 21

Poland syndrome 17, 137
Polydactyly 77, 137
Popliteal pterygium 88
Position of non-ossified capital epiphysis 105f
Postural and congenital deformities of foot and ankle 73
Proximal femoral focal deficiency 63, 63f
Pseudochondroplasia 20
Pterygia syndrome 88, 93
Pterygium syndrome 21

R
Radial club hand 131, 132f
　deformity 131
Reconstructive surgery 47
Reduction of dislocation 102
Reflected head of rectus femoris tendon 102
Renal
　agenesis 134
　dysplasia 17
Rheumatic disorders manifesting in neonatal period 160
Rubella 17
Rubinstein-Taybi syndrome 21, 138, 156

S
Sacrococcygeal teratoma 161, 162
Scalp defect 156
Septic arthritis 142, 144f
Severe rhizomelic type 170
Shenton's line 105f
Shoulder girdle anomalies 123
Siamese twins 163
Skin and soft tissue injuries 38
Skull 6
　fractures 39
Smith-Lemli-Pitz syndrome 155
Spina bifida 114
Spinal defects 114
Splaying of metaphyses of bones around knees 23f
Spondyloepiphyseal dysplasia 20, 21
　congenita 14, 20, 21, 25
Spontaneous correction of kyphoscoliosis of tibia fibular bone growth 52f
Sprengel's shoulder 123
Staphylococcus aureus 142, 146, 148
Sticklar's syndrome 20
Straight X-ray 103
Straightening of short tibia 46f

Streeter syndrome 47, 137
Syme's amputation 65
Symphalangism 76
Syndactyly 76, 137
Syphilis 17
Systemic lupus erythematosus 160

T
Terminal deficiencies 46
Tetanus immune globulin 152
Tetralogy of Fallot 134
Thanatophoric dwarfism 14, 20, 21, 24
Thomsen's disease 33, 34
Thorax 7
Thorough examination of baby 11
Thrombocytopenia-absent radius syndrome 156
Tibial agenesis 58
Toxoplasmosis 17
Treacher Collins syndrome 20, 155
Turner syndrome 15
Types of
　arthrogryposis 89
　disorders of voluntary muscles 33
　osteotomies 69
　syndactyly 137

U
Upper limb 7, 123

V
Vascular insufficiency 17
Velocardiofacial syndrome 155
Ventricular septal defect 134
Vertebral
　agenesis 113-115
　anomalies 113
　column 7
Vitamin D resistant rickets 15

W
Walker-Warburg syndrome 154
Whistling face syndrome 21
Widervanck or Cervico-oculo-acoustic syndrome 155

X
X-linked
　dominant inheritance 15
　recessive inheritance 14

Z
Z-plasty 122, 139